DATE DUE

MAR 1 7 1994	OCT 1 7 1996
MAR 3 1 1994	OCT 3 1 1996
OCT 2 6 1994	FEB 2 7 1997
NOV - 7 1994	OCT 2 9 1998
NOV 1 4 1994	SEP 2 5 2001
NOV 2 8 1994	OCT 2 9 2001
DEC 1 2 1994	
JAN - 4 1995	
JAN 1 9 1995	
MAR 2 1 1995	
OCT 1 0 1995	
OCT 3 1 1995	
NOV 1 8 1995	
JAN 1 9 1996	
FEB 1 6 1996	
MAR 1 6 1996	
OCT - 3 1996	

ATHEROSCLEROSIS REVIEWS
Volume 22

Triglycerides
The Role in Diabetes and Atherosclerosis

Atherosclerosis Reviews

Chief Editors: Antonio M. Gotto and Rodolfo Paoletti

INTERNATIONAL ADVISORY BOARD

Atherosclerosis Reviews
Volume 22

Triglycerides
The Role in Diabetes and Atherosclerosis

Editors

Antonio M. Gotto, Jr., M.D.
Department of Medicine
The Methodist Hospital
Baylor College of Medicine
Houston, Texas

Rodolfo Paoletti, M.D.
Institute of Pharmacological
Sciences
University of Milan
Milan, Italy

Raven Press New York

Raven Press, 1185 Avenue of the Americas, New York, New York 10036

Made in the United States of America

Library of Congress Cataloging-in-Publication Data

Triglycerides: the role in diabetes and atherosclerosis/editors,
    Antonio M. Gotto, Rodolfo Paoletti.
        p.   cm.—(Atherosclerosis reviews: v. 22)
    Proceedings of an international symposium held in Vienna, Austria,
May 23–26, 1990.
    Includes bibliographical references and index.
    ISBN 0-88167-813-9
    1. Hypertriglyceridemia—Congresses.   2. Atherosclerosis—
Pathophysiology—Congresses.   3. Coronary heart disease—
Pathophysiology—Congresses.   4. Diabetes—Complications and
sequelae—Congresses.   I. Gotto, Antonio M.   II. Paoletti, Rodolfo.
III. Series
    [DNLM: 1. Atherosclerosis—metabolism—congresses.   2. Diabetes
Mellitus—metabolism—congresses.   3. Triglycerides—metabolism—
congresses.   QU 85 T828 1990]
    RC692.A729   vol. 22
    [RC632.H888]
    616.1'36 s—dc20
    [616.1'36]
    DNLM/DLC
    for Library of Congress   91-15565
                                                                                CIP

9 8 7 6 5 4 3 2

Contents

Preface

Triglycerides are once again in the medical foreground. In the late 1950s and early 1960s, the subject was one of considerable emphasis. The mid-1970s saw the "rediscovery of high-density lipoprotein (HDL) triglycerides" and thus a tendency to discount triglycerides as a risk factor for coronary heart disease (CHD). In 1980, Stephen Hulley and colleagues questioned the rationale of measuring triglycerides as a cardiovascular risk factor [*New England Journal of Medicine* (302:1383–1389)]. The adult treatment guidelines of the National Cholesterol Education Program, published in 1988, barely recognized hypertriglyceridemia. This panel endorsed the recommendations of the National Institutes of Health's 1984 consensus conference on triglycerides, but in its algorithm for evaluating hypercholesterolemia used triglycerides only for calculating the low-density lipoprotein (LDL) cholesterol value.

In the Framingham Heart Study, serum triglyceride concentration was found to be an independent predictor of CHD risk in women but not in men. Hypertriglyceridemia has been thought to be important as a risk factor, notably in patients with familial combined hyperlipidema, dysbetalipoproteinemia, renal failure or chronic renal disease, and especially in patients with diabetes. Patients with CHD and survivors of myocardial infarction have almost invariably, as groups, had higher triglyceride levels than comparison groups.

It is generally agreed that there are stronger data relating LDL cholesterol and CHD than triglycerides and CHD. On univariate analysis, serum triglyceride concentration is usually a predictor of CHD, but much of the significance is lost on multivariate analysis. The HDL level, which is inversely related to the triglyceride concentration, corrects for a significant part of the CHD risk attributed to serum triglycerides. However, some statisticians and epidemiologists question the appropriateness of multivariate analyses of such closely related, interdependent variables.

With the renewed interest in hypertriglyceridemia, the metabolism of the triglyceride-rich lipoproteins is under intense investigation in a broad range of areas. There is considerable evidence that triglyceride-rich remnant lipoproteins are atherogenic. Also, postprandial lipemia has been linked with increased CHD risk, bearing out D. Zilversmit's early prediction of an atherogenic role for the partially metabolized dietary fat particle. In several populations, at least 25% of people with early CHD have total cholesterol levels below 200 mg/dl, but they also demonstrate elevations of triglycerides and low concentrations of HDL cholesterol, in particular HDL_2.

Melissa Austin of the University of Washington (Seattle) and her colleagues have studied hypertriglyceridemia using both epidemiologic and familial approaches. They have identified an LDL subclass pattern that is characterized by a predominance of small, dense LDL particles and that correlates with a threefold-increased CHD risk, elevated concentrations of intermediate-density lipoprotein cholesterol, very-low-density lipoprotein cholesterol, triglycerides, and low concentrations of HDL and HDL_2. The dense-LDL pattern occurs in familial combined hyperlipidemia and is also described in syndrome X, which is thought to be related to insulin resistance and hyperinsulinemia. The same set of metabolic parameters appears to be present in dyslipidemic hypertension and in the hyper-apoB syndrome described by earlier investigators.

Over the past 2 years, an international committee has been working to develop a new consensus document on the evaluation and treatment of hypertriglyceridemia. Publication is anticipated sometime in 1991. This volume of *Atherosclerosis Reviews* should provide enough perspective to enable the physician or researcher to understand the new developments in the fields of hypertriglyceridemia and diabetes. It clarifies not only basic research findings but also the implications of that research for the practice of medicine.

Antonio M. Gotto, Jr., M.D., D.Phil.

Acknowledgment

This volume presents the proceedings of the International Symposium titled Triglycerides—The Role in Diabetes and Atherosclerosis held in Vienna, Austria, May 23–26, 1990. The symposium was made possible by an educational grant from Farmitalia Carlo Erba—Erbamont Group, Milan, Italy.

Introduction

For the first time, the role of triglycerides was the central issue of an international conference (Vienna, 1990). This revival of interest is based on the most recent biochemical and epidemiological investigations; the field is now at the threshold of a new therapeutic era, with specific drugs acting with a well-established mode of action. The meeting—on which this volume of *Atherosclerosis Reviews* is based—covered most aspects of triglyceride research and clinical science.

Triglyceride metabolism is discussed in detail under normal (Olivecrona) and pathological conditions (Shepard, Gianturco, Ginsberg), with particular emphasis on the role of insulin and other hormones (Steiner, Knopp) and in diabetes (Pometta). Particular emphasis also is given to the sometimes elusive relationship between triglyceride atherosclerosis, as shown by the Framingham (Wilson) and Helsinki studies (Manninen), and the present evidence on the connection with coronary heart disease (Austin, Hamsten, Galton). Triglycerides also are related to peripheral (Olsson) and to the atherosclerosis vascular consequences of diabetes.

The emerging relationship between plasma triglycerides, fibrinolysis, and Lp(a) are reviewed by Tremoli, Kostner, and Rosseneu, respectively. The role of triglycerides is also present in the insulin-resistance syndrome and in the more complex syndrome including hypertension, insulin resistance, and lipoprotein alterations.

The therapeutic approach to hypertriglyceridemias is reported in detail. Diet is the first approach (Nestel), particularly if combined with exercise (Wood), and several classes of drugs, such as fibrates, bignamides, and nicotinic acid have clinical use. Acipimox, an analogue of nicotinic acid (Walldius) extensively tested in diabetic hyperlipidemia (Alberti), is discussed for its efficacy (Barter, Scott) and safety (Buckley). The effects of bile acid sequestrants in relation to triglyceride metabolism are also discussed (Ericsson).

This volume contains a critical state-of-the-art review of our knowledge in this field of clinical and biological interest. Triglycerides are clearly emerging as cardiovascular risk factors, and the theoretical basis and available means for their control are presented comprehensively for the first time in a publication that will certainly stimulate new investigations and be of interest not only to cardiovascular experts but also to diabetologists and internists.

Rodolfo Paoletti, M.D.

Atherosclerosis Reviews, Volume 22,
edited by A. M. Gotto, Jr. and R. Paoletti.
Raven Press, Ltd., New York © 1991.

Metabolic Consequences of Hypertriglyceridemia

James Shepherd and Christopher J. Packard

Institute of Biochemistry, Royal Infirmary, Glasgow G4 OSF, Scotland

More than 95% of the triglyceride (TG) that circulates through the human bloodstream does so in association with chylomicrons produced in the intestine or very-low-density lipoproteins (VLDL) secreted by the liver. The ease with which we are able to handle these TG-rich particles has a profound influence on the structure, metabolism, and function of cholesterol-enriched low- and high-density lipoproteins (LDL, HDL). This chapter discusses the interrelationships among the plasma lipoproteins, focusing on the role of TG in modulating their metabolism and influencing their propensity to promote atherosclerosis.

EXOGENOUS TRIGLYCERIDE METABOLISM

Following its absorption in the intestine (Fig. 1), dietary fat is packaged into large TG-rich chylomicron particles that contain on their surface a number of apolipoproteins (apoA-I, apoA-IV, $apoB_{48}$) that direct and regulate their metabolism. Elaboration of these particles is critically dependent on the production of apoB. In the intestine, this process involves a unique mRNA editing process (1).

The human genome contains only a single copy of the human apoB gene. In the liver, the gene is fully expressed (generating $apoB_{100}$). However, intestinal deamidation of the apoB messenger introduces a stop codon (a CAA → UAA conversion), truncating the apoB to a 2152 amino acid product ($apoB_{48}$). Although the biological benefits inherent in this process are not clear, it is possible that this mechanism alters the metabolism of particles containing B_{48} by eliminating their ability to bind to the LDL receptor and redirecting their catabolism into alternative degradative pathways.

When the chylomicrons appear in the plasma, they acquire apoE and apoC proteins from HDL and have a density <0.95 g/ml. ApoC-II modulates lipolysis of the chylomicron by acting as a cofactor for lipoprotein lipase located on capillary endothelial surfaces in skeletal muscle and adipose tissue (2). This enzyme, which is under strong hormonal control, promotes hydrolysis of TG from the particle core, releasing fatty acids for storage or

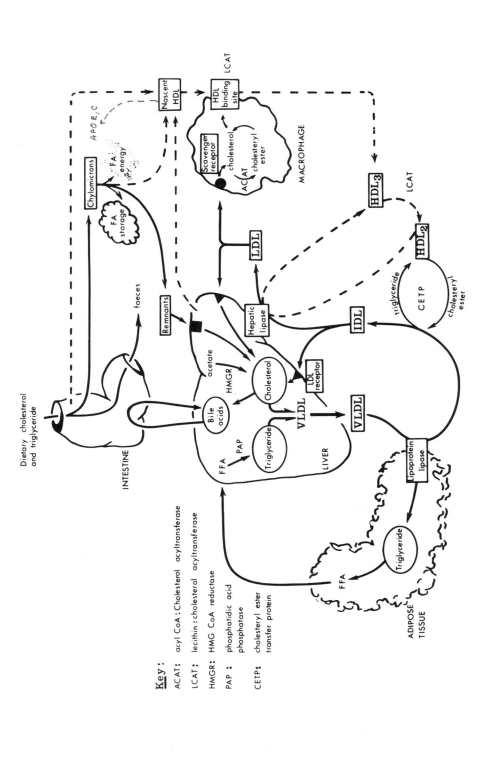

Key:

ACAT: acyl CoA:Cholesterol acyltransferase

LCAT: lecithin:cholesterol acyltransferase

HMGR: HMG CoA reductase

PAP : phosphatidic acid phosphatase

CETP: cholesteryl ester transfer protein

energy requirements. The chylomicron itself shrinks progressively, shedding its surface phospholipid and small molecular weight proteins into the HDL density interval, to leave a remnant which by virtue of the apoE on its surface is cleared rapidly by the parenchymal cells of the liver. These cells have an LDL receptor–like polypeptide (LDL receptor-related protein or LRP) that has all the properties expected of the putative chylomicron receptor (3). It binds apoE but not apoB and is insensitive to sterol regulation. In this regard, the apoE phenotype of an individual has a strong impact on his or her ability to clear chylomicron remnant particles. The presence of E_2, even in a single dose, significantly retards chylomicron remnant clearance.

Recent studies have suggested that coronary artery disease (CAD) may be associated with a relative inability to clear chylomicron remnants efficiently from the circulation (4). Administration of a TG-enriched meal to individuals with angiographically proven CAD (Fig. 2) revealed that these subjects metabolized TG-rich lipoprotein (TGRLP) particles less efficiently than age-matched healthy controls. Interestingly, the fasting plasma lipid and lipoprotein levels (Table 1) were also significantly different from those of the control subjects. In particular, their circulating LDL cholesterol values were 24% higher and their HDL cholesterol 17% lower than the CAD-negative individuals. The reduction in HDL affected both subfractions. The masses of HDL_2 and HDL_3 in the blood of the ischemic subjects were 30% and 14% less than in the controls, respectively. Nonlipid risk factors like blood pressure and Quetelet's index did not show any differences between the groups. These observations raise the interesting possibility that defects in the handling of triglyceride-rich particles might be linked to alterations in the metabolism of LDL and HDL.

ENDOGENOUS TRIGLYCERIDE METABOLISM

The two-step chylomicron clearance pathway delivers TG and cholesterol to the liver, where it may be stored or resecreted as components of endog-

---

FIG. 1 Lipoprotein metabolism. Following absorption, dietary fat is packaged into large triglyceride(TG)-rich chylomicron particles within the enterocyte and secreted into the circulation. There, lipolysis reduces the particle's TG core and makes redundant part of its surface coat, which is shed to high-density lipoprotein (HDL). The remnants produced in the process are rapidly assimilated by a receptor-mediated mechanism in the liver. In the fasting state, very-low-density lipoproteins replace chylomicrons as the major TG transporters, and the liver dominates lipoprotein metabolism. Cholesterol and TG elaborated in this organ are incorporated into VLDL, which are released into the plasma. There they become subject to tissue lipolysis, which degrades them to low-density lipoproteins (LDL) via an intermediate species (IDL). The LDL is removed by receptors on the liver and peripheral tissues. When these are saturated, an alternative, scavenger pathway becomes dominant. Interchange of lipids between circulating lipoprotein particles is facilitated by the plasma enzymes lecithin: cholesterol acyltransferase and cholesteryl ester transfer protein, both of which participate in the process of reverse cholesterol transport from peripheral sites to the liver, where the sterol is excreted. ACAT, acyl CoA: cholesterol acyltransferase; LCAT, lecithin: cholesterol acyltransferase; HMGR, HMG CoA reductase; PAP, phosphatidic acid phosphatase; CETP, cholesteryl ester transfer protein.

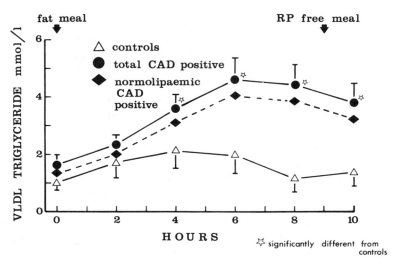

FIG. 2. Postprandial lipidemia in coronary artery disease. Thirty-four coronary artery disease (CAD)-positive and 18 CAD-negative subjects were fed a standard fat meal. The flux of triglyceride (TG) through their d < 1.006 kg/1 lipoproteins was followed over a 24-hr period. Peak TG values in the 4-, 6-, and 8-hr serum samples after fat feeding were significantly higher ($p < 0.05$) in the CAD-positive group. This difference persisted even when lipoprotein values from hypercholesterolemic subjects were eliminated from the CAD-positive group.

enous lipoproteins. This organ also participates (Fig. 1) in the continuous elaboration of TG-rich VLDL particles that lie within the density range of 0.95–1.006 g/ml. These particles contain $apoB_{100}$, apoC, and apoE on their surface and are subject to the same hydrolytic process as the chylomicrons. Lipolysis here results in the production of a relatively cholesteryl ester–rich intermediate-density remnant lipoprotein particle (IDL, d = 1.006–1.019 g/ml). In normal individuals, about one-half of these remnants are cleared directly by the liver; the remainder continue down the delipidation cascade to form LDL (d = 1.019–1.063 g/ml), the major cholesterol transporter in human plasma.

Studies of human lipase deficiency syndromes have shown that lipolysis of large TG-rich VLDL to smaller remnants is dependent entirely on the activity of lipoprotein lipase whereas the conversion of IDL to LDL requires the intervention of hepatic lipase, a second enzyme located on the membranes of liver parenchymal cells. These two enzymes, from distinct but related genes, are particularly important not only in modulating TG transport through the plasma but also in influencing the structure and metabolism of the denser cholesterol-rich lipoproteins, LDL and HDL. Individuals with high lipoprotein lipase activity (such as young women or athletes) have particularly active lipoprotein lipase, low VLDL triglyceride concentrations,

TABLE 1. *Coronary risk factors in CAD-negative and CAD-positive subjects*

Parameter	CAD-negative group ($n = 18$)	CAD-positive ($n = 34$)	Significance[a]
Age (yr)	49.6 ± 9.0	51.7 ± 6.6	NS
Systolic blood pressure (mm Hg)	125 ± 15	126 ± 12	NS
Diastolic blood pressure (mm Hg)	74 ± 12	79 ± 10	NS
Queletet index	25.6 ± 4.0	26.8 ± 3.0	NS
Plasma cholesterol (mmol/L)	6.11 ± 0.96	6.91 ± 1.34	< 0.02
Plasma triglyceride (mmol/L)	2.09 ± 0.96	2.52 ± 0.96	NS
LDL cholesterol (mmol/L)	3.98 ± 0.85	4.89 ± 1.22	< 0.01
HDL cholesterol (mmol/L)	1.18 ± 0.27	0.98 ± 0.24	< 0.01
HDL$_2$ mass (mg/dl)	46 ± 26	32 ± 14	< 0.05
HDL$_3$ mass (mg/dl)	249 ± 42	213 ± 41	< 0.01

CAD, coronary artery disease.
[a] Unpaired *t* test or Mann-Whitney analysis.

and high HDL (particularly HDL$_2$) concentrations. This reflects the metabolic relationship between TG-rich particle metabolism and HDL. Conversely, the higher hepatic lipase activities found in men and in exaggerated form in individuals taking anabolic steroids result in low HDL values. Therefore, the ratio of lipoprotein/hepatic lipase activity may offer a strong indication of atherosclerosis risk.

The important role played by hepatic lipase in the metabolism of LDL and HDL is clearly evident in individuals hereditarily deficient in this enzyme (5). They are completely unable to convert IDL to LDL and HDL$_2$ to HDL$_3$ (Fig. 3); the HDL that accumulates in their plasma is large and TG-rich (Table 2), reflecting their continuous acquisition of TG from VLDL in exchange for cholesterol ester. This process is mediated by cholesterol ester transfer protein (CETP). Its effects (Fig. 4) are normally balanced by the actions of hepatic lipase, which rapidly hydrolyzes the TG present in HDL$_2$ to produce smaller and denser HDL$_3$. Individuals who lack either the CETP gene (6) or are completely deficient (7) in TG-rich particles (i.e., who are abetablipoproteinemic), accumulate HDL$_2$ enriched in cholesterol ester rather than TG.

TRIGLYCERIDE-RICH PARTICLES AND ATHEROGENESIS

The VLDL elaborated by the liver (Fig. 1) varies in size and composition in different individuals depending on its relative proportions of TG and apoB$_{100}$. Kinetic studies (8) have shown that large VLDL (such as that secreted by diabetics or induced by carbohydrate-loading) are hydrolyzed to remnants that are cleared directly from the circulation without contributing to the LDL pool. Smaller, cholesterol-enriched VLDL particles are the main source of these remnants.

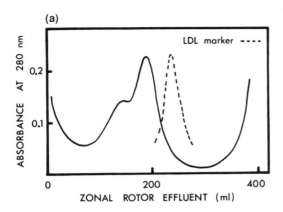

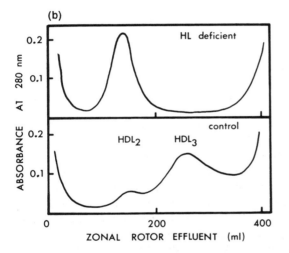

FIG. 3. Effects of hepatic lipase deficiency on plasma (**a**) low-density lipoproteins (LDL) and (**b**) high-density lipoproteins (HDL). Rate zonal ultracentrifugation of LDL (a) and HDL (b) from a patient with hepatic lipase deficiency and a healthy control subject. The hepatic lipase defect is associated with the presence in the circulation of more buoyant cholesterol-rich lipoproteins.

Lipase deficiency states produce extreme examples of disrupted TG-rich particle metabolism. However, less florid changes are also seen in familial hypercholesterolemic subjects who lack the classical LDL receptor or in type III hyperlipoproteinemic individuals who have inherited a mutation in apoE that compromises its ability to interact with its receptor. Both of these conditions are characterized by (a) accumulation of cholesterol ester–rich VLDL remnants and IDL in the circulation and (b) inhibited conversion of IDL to LDL. They are further characterized by a greatly increased predisposition to coronary artery disease. These factors suggest that particular subclasses of TG-rich lipoproteins may predispose the individual to atherosclerosis. Further credence is lent this hypothesis by the fact that these remnant particles are the only naturally occurring plasma lipoproteins that can induce cholesterol ester accumulation in cultured macrophages (9).

TABLE 2. *Plasma lipoproteins in hepatic lipase deficiency*

	Total	VLDL	LDL	HDL
Cholesterol[a]	5.10 ± 1.05	0.75 ± 0.41	2.18 ± 0.29	1.96 ± 0.25
Triglyceride[a]	2.82 ± 0.49	0.66 ± 0.31	1.42 ± 0.39	0.64 ± 0.40
C/T ratio		1.1	1.5	3.1
10–90 Percentile C/T ratio		0.4–0.8	6.0–16.0	5.0–16.3

[a] mmol/L

Although these data point to a direct role for TG-rich lipoproteins in the pathogenesis of atherosclerosis, these particles may also promote the risk for disease in more subtle, indirect ways (10). Individuals with sustained hypertriglyceridemia exhibit higher CETP activity in their plasma. This protein promotes the rapid molecular exchange of cholesteryl ester for TG between all lipoprotein species in the bloodstream. When an excess of TG-rich lipoproteins is present, the Law of Mass Action drives the equilibrium toward TG enrichment in HDL with concomitant cholesteryl ester accumulation in VLDL. The latter may then promote delivery of cholesteryl ester to macrophages. At the same time, TG enrichment of the HDL particle makes it a good substrate for hepatic lipase, which hydrolyzes it to smaller, denser species that are cleared more rapidly from the bloodstream. The net effect is to lower circulating HDL levels and compromise the process of reverse cholesterol transport.

A similar phenomenon occurs within the LDL density spectrum. Here, higher plasma TG levels, even within the reference range, skew the distribution of LDL particles toward smaller, denser species that, on the basis of epidemiological studies, are linked to increased risk of coronary heart disease (11,12). Indeed, there appears to be a risk syndrome, common in

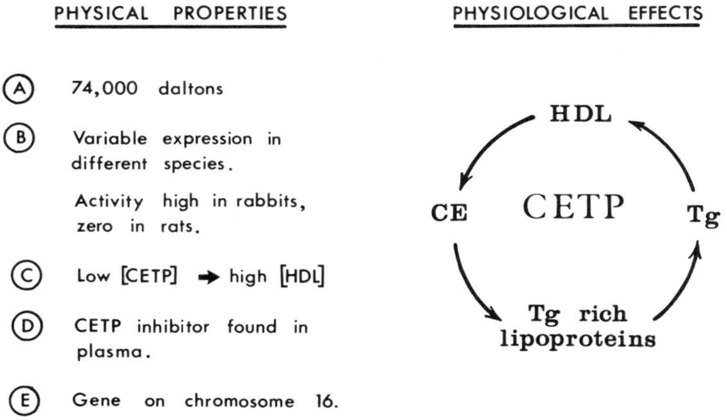

PHYSICAL PROPERTIES   PHYSIOLOGICAL EFFECTS

(A) 74,000 daltons

(B) Variable expression in different species.

Activity high in rabbits, zero in rats.

(C) Low [CETP] → high [HDL]

(D) CETP inhibitor found in plasma.

(E) Gene on chromosome 16.

FIG. 4. Properties and functions of cholesteryl ester transfer protein.

the population, characterized by the constellation (13) of moderate hypertriglyceridemia, low HDL_2, and small, dense LDL. Although the metabolic relationships that link raised plasma TG levels to risk for coronary heart disease are becoming more clearly understood, further investigation is needed before they can be credited with the same importance now attributed to raised blood cholesterol levels.

A growing body of evidence indicates that TG-rich particles contribute directly to the atherogenic process. Macrophages have been shown to bind and internalize TG-rich particles in proportion to their apoE content (14); they also possess on their membranes a binding domain that does not require apoE but instead appears to recognize peroxidized lipoproteins (15). Assimilation of these species stimulates cholesterol esterification at twice the rate seen during uptake of unoxidized lipoproteins.

REFERENCES

1. Powell LM, Wallis SC, Pease RJ, Edwards YH, Knott TJ, Scott J. A novel form of tissue specific RNA processing produces apolipoprotein B48 in intestine. *Cell* 1987;50:831–840.
2. Breckenridge WC, Little JA, Steiner G, Chow A, Poapst M. Hypertriglyceridemia associated with deficiency of apolipoprotein CII. *N Engl J Med* 1978;298:1265–1273.
3. Beisiegel U, Weber W, Ihrke G, Hirz J, Stanley KK. The LDL receptor related protein. LRP is an apolipoprotein E binding protein. *Nature* 1989;341:162–164.
4. Simpson HS, Williamson CM, Pringle S, et al. Hypolipidemic drugs and chylomicron metabolism. In: Windler E, Greten H, eds. *Intestinal lipid and lipoprotein metabolism* Munchen: W Zuckschwerdt Verlag: 194–201.
5. Demant T, Carlson LA, Holmquist L, et al. Lipoprotein metabolism in hepatic lipase deficiency: studies on the turnover of apolipoprotein B and on the effect of hepatic lipase on high density lipoprotein. *J Lipid Res* 1988; 29:1603–1611.
6. Koizumi J, Mabuchi H, Yoshimura A, et al. Deficiency of serum cholesteryl ester transfer activity in patients with familial hyperalphalipoproteinemia. *Atherosclerosis* 1985; 58:175–186.
7. Scanu AM, Aggerbeck LP, Kruski AW, Lim CT, Kayden HJ. A study of the abnormal lipoproteins in abetalipoproteinemia. *J Clin Invest* 1974;53:440–453.
8. Packard CJ, Munro A, Lorimer AR, Gotto AM, Shepherd J. Metabolism of apolipoprotein B in large triglyceride-rich VLDL of normal and hypertriglyceridemic subjects. *J Clin Invest* 1984;74:2178–2192.
9. Gianturco SH, Bradley WA, Gotto AM, Morrisett JD, Peavy DL. Hypertriglyceridemic VLDL induce triglyceride synthesis and accumulation in mouse peritoneal macrophages. *J Clin Invest* 1982;70:168–178.
10. Deckelbaum RJ, Granot E, Oschry Y, Rose L, Eisenberg S. Plasma triglyceride determines structure—composition in low and high density lipoproteins. *Arteriosclerosis* 1984;4:226–231.
11. Krauss RM. Relationship of intermediate and low density lipoprotein subspecies to risk of coronary artery disease. *Am Heart J* 1987;113:578–582.
12. Austin MA. Plasma triglyceride as a risk factor for coronary heart disease. *Am J Epidemiol* 1989;129:249–259.
13. Breier C, Patsch JR, Michelberger V, Drexel H, Knapp E, Braunsteiner H. Risk factors for coronary artery disease: a study comparing hypercholesterolaemia and hypertriglyceridaemia in angiographically characterised patients. *Eur J Clin Invest* 1989;19:419–423.
14. Bates SR, Coughlin BA, Mazzone T, Borensztajn J, Getz GS. Apoprotein E mediates the interaction of VLDL with macrophages. *J Lipid Res* 1987;28:787–797.
15. Parthasarathy S, Quinn MT, Schwerke DC, Carew TE, Steinberg D. Oxidative modification of VLDL. *Arteriosclerosis* 1989;9:398–404.

Atherosclerosis Reviews, Volume 22,
edited by A. M. Gotto, Jr. and R. Paoletti.
Raven Press, Ltd., New York © 1991.

A Cellular Basis for the Atherogenicity of Triglyceride-Rich Lipoproteins

Sandra H. Gianturco and William A. Bradley

*Department of Medicine, University of Alabama at Birmingham,
Birmingham, Alabama, 35294*

Initiation of atherosclerosis is thought to involve, among other factors, abnormal cellular uptake of lipoproteins leading to foam cell formation (1) and injury of the endothelium (2). To identify potential mechanisms that would explain the association of hypertriglyceridemia with atherosclerosis, we conducted a series of studies demonstrating that certain triglyceride-rich lipoproteins (TGRLP) bind abnormally to cellular receptors. Consequently, they convert macrophages into foam cells and cause endothelial cell dysfunction *in vitro*. This process suggests that these TGRLP are highly atherogenic (3–12).

TGRLP are heterogeneous in origin, structure, interactions with cellular lipoprotein receptors, and potential atherogenicity. They are synthesized in both the liver and the intestine. Hepatically derived TGRLP [very-low-density lipoproteins (VLDL), d < 1.006 g/ml, S_f 20–400] are present in the postabsorptive as well as the postprandial state.

Intestinally derived TGRLP, chylomicrons and their remnants, carry dietary cholesterol and triglyceride (TG) and contain $apoB_{48}$ rather than the $apoB_{100}$ characteristic of hepatically derived VLDL. Intestinally derived TGRLP are normally present only in the postprandial state, but $apoB_{48}$ is detected in VLDL in the postabsorptive state in most hypertriglyceridemic subjects (3), and chylomicrons are present in some hypertriglyceridemic subjects, particularly in those with diabetes (13).

An important characteristic of TGRLP that is often overlooked is that each large TGRLP particle carries more cholesterol and cholesteryl ester than does one low-density lipoprotein (LDL) particle (14). Because compositions are often expressed as percentages, and the percentage of cholesterol plus cholesteryl ester in LDL is near 50% and only 10% in VLDL S_f 100 to 400 (VLDL$_1$), it is erroneously assumed that LDL contain more sterol than VLDL. The mass of each TGRLP particle is far greater than that of LDL (chylomicrons M_r ~500 × 10^6; VLDL$_1$ ~30 × 10^6; and only 2.2 × 10^6 for LDL), and this difference in mass/particle translates into far more

9

molecules of cholesterol and cholesteryl ester per particle in the large TGRLP than in LDL. For example, one chylomicron particle ($S_f > 400$) carries approximately 60,000 molecules of cholesterol plus cholesteryl ester, one VLDL S_f 100–400 carries ~10,000, and one LDL carries only ~2,000 total sterol molecules (14).

In addition, each of the TGRLP carries an enormous number of TG molecules (~24,000 in $VLDL_1$ and 500,000 in chylomicrons versus only 300 in LDL) (14). When the data are expressed in these terms, it is easier to accept the notion that TGRLP could be atherogenic (i.e., deliver excess cholesterol to monocyte-macrophages or cells of the artery wall) if they could be taken up by the cells. It even seems reasonable to speculate that these particles could be more atherogenic than LDL, because one chylomicron could deliver 30 times and a $VLDL_1$ five times as much cholesterol as could one LDL particle. In addition, the TGRLP could deliver massive levels of TG that, if hydrolyzed intracellularly, could produce toxic levels of fatty acids. In an earlier article, we suggested that this was the basis for the toxicity of HTG-VLDL toward cultured endothelial cells (6).

Fortunately, not all TGRLP have rapid, receptor-mediated access to cells. Large normal VLDL (S_f 60–400) from fasting normal subjects do not bind to the LDL receptor (4,5,7) and do not cause rapid, receptor-mediated lipid engorgement in macrophages (8). Small normal VLDL S_f 20–60 can bind to the LDL receptor (5,7) but do not cause lipid-loading in macrophages (8).

By contrast, TGRLP from hypertriglyceridemic subjects are abnormal in composition, distribution, and cellular interactions, and are potentially atherogenic. Indeed, chylomicrons and large VLDL ($S_f > 100$) from certain hypertriglyceridemic subjects are the only native human lipoproteins that can cause, without modification *in vitro*, rapid, receptor-mediated lipid engorgement in monocyte-macrophages, causing foam cell morphology within 4 hr *in vitro* (8).

Moreover, HTG-$VLDL_1$ but not normal $VLDL_1$ not only deliver cholesterol to cultured endothelial cells but are toxic to the cells (6) or induce giant cell formation (unpublished observations with F. Booyse). These are potentially atherogenic cellular consequences of receptor-mediated uptake of abnormal TGRLP, since in the arterial wall giant cells and denuded areas are sites of monocyte and platelet attachment.

In fasting normal subjects, approximately 75% of the total VLDL (d < 1.006 g/ml) are small (S_f 20–60) and similar to intermediate-density lipoproteins (IDL) in composition and cellular interactions (relatively TG-poor and cholesteryl ester–rich and bind to the LDL receptor via apoB) (3). By contrast, in most subjects with hypertriglyceridemia, large VLDL, $S_f > 60$, comprise the bulk of the total VLDL. Thus, to compare total VLDL from normal subjects with total VLDL from hypertriglyceridemic subjects, as has been done in some studies, is to compare very different populations because of the different cellular interactions of large versus small normal VLDL.

Consistent with the *in vitro* studies, *in vivo* turnover studies indicate that in normal subjects a large proportion of small VLDL are catabolized directly and are not converted into LDL (15). Turnover studies in hypertriglyceridemic subjects indicate that even large VLDL are lost from the plasma compartment (15), most likely by receptor-mediated routes.

The abnormal TGRLP found in hypertriglyceridemic subjects could be considered to be VLDL modified *in vivo*. HTG-VLDL subclasses have more apoE and more $apoB_{48}$ and apoB fragments than comparable normal VLDL subfractions (3). The additional apoE of large fasting HTG-VLDL (S_f 60–400) is in a conformation different from the apoE present in normal VLDL S_f 60–400. The "extra" apoE, in sharp contrast to the apoE of normal VLDL, binds to the LDL receptor (3,9), is cleavable by thrombin (3,9), and is accessible to the anti-apoE monoclonal antibody 1D7, which recognizes the receptor binding domain of apoE (unpublished observations). Large normal VLDL $S_f > 60$, which do not bind to LDL receptors (4,5,7), acquire the ability to bind after incubation with exogenous apoE and then resemble HTG-VLDL (7,16). The extra apoE in large HTG-VLDL is in an accessible conformation, unlike the inaccessible apoE of large normal VLDL; accessible apoE mediates binding to the LDL receptor (3,9). We speculated that in hypertriglyceridemic subjects, this accessible apoE transfers into VLDL during its prolonged residence time in plasma, analogous to addition of exogenous apoE *in vitro* to normal VLDL (9). We further suggested that the apoE of large normal VLDL represents endogenous apoE, synthesized and packaged with VLDL in the liver (9).

Abnormal uptake of HTG-VLDL by the LDL receptor could be atherogenic, since LDL receptors are expressed on all cells, including cells of the artery wall, such as endothelial cells and smooth muscle cells.

Macrophage uptake of abnormal, modified VLDL and chylomicrons, however, appears to be mediated primarily by a receptor that we refer to as the "modified VLDL" receptor, which is distinct from both the LDL receptor and the acetyl LDL receptor. This receptor is present on human monocytes as well as on differentiated macrophages but not on human fibroblasts (11). Uptake of TGRLP by the modified VLDL receptor of macrophages results in massive lipid engorgement, both TG and cholesteryl ester (10,11). The receptor is distinct from the LDL receptor immunochemically, in ligand specificity (apoE is not required for binding), in distribution (only in cells of reticuloendothelial origin), and in regulation (it is not regulated by cellular sterol content) (11). Moreover, the modified VLDL receptor, unlike the acetyl LDL receptor or the LDL receptor, is not affected by state of differentiation in human THP-1 monocyte-macrophages (12). The macrophage plasma membrane proteins that are likely modified VLDL receptor candidates differ from the LDL receptor immunochemically (11). These proteins differ from other lipoprotein receptors in apparent molecular weight (11,12).

In hypertriglyceridemia, $apoB_{48}$ is often found in VLDL; in some subjects, fragmented $apoB_{100}$ also appears in the VLDL density range. TGRLP containing these apoB species bind to the modified VLDL macrophage receptor, whereas normal VLDL containing $apoB_{100}$ do not (11,12). Proteolysis of VLDL that eliminates immunochemically detectable apoE and cleaves apoB into large fragments enhances binding to the macrophage receptor (11). Taken together, these studies indicate that apoE is not required for binding to the modified VLDL receptor and suggest that an apoB domain accessible in TGRLP particles containing $apoB_{48}$ or $apoB_{100}$ fragments mediates binding.

Thus, the binding determinants of uptake of abnormal VLDL by the LDL receptor and the macrophage receptor for modified VLDL are distinct. The LDL receptor requires apoE of a particular conformation. The modified VLDL receptor does not require apoE but appears to require a domain of apoB accessible in chylomicrons and certain HTG-VLDL that may be inaccessible in normal VLDL or LDL.

Preliminary observations with postprandial TGRLP subspecies from normal and hypertriglyceridemic subjects support Zilversmit's hypothesis that postprandial TGRLP can be atherogenic (17). Using a fat load composed of eggs, cheese, toast, and milk, as described by Weintraub et al. (18), we have studied the changes in atherogenicity and structure and amounts of TGRLP subspecies postprandially. The total TGRLP were subfractionated by cumulative flotation into classes of $S_f > 400$, S_f 100–400, 60–100, and 20–60. Immunochemical blots demonstrate that all TGRLP subspecies from normal subjects acquire extra apoE that is accessible to cleavage by thrombin at 2–6 hr postprandially. Consistent with this compositional change, postprandial TGRLP subspecies S_f 60–400 acquire the ability to bind to LDL receptors, as detected both by ligand blotting studies and fibroblast uptake studies. In addition, $apoB_{48}$ is present in all postprandial TGRLP subspecies (even in the S_f 20–60 range). Ligand blots indicate that postprandial TGRLP show enhanced binding to the macrophage-modified VLDL receptor protein candidates. In normal subjects, only the $S_f > 400$ subfraction caused significant rapid (i.e., 4 hr incubations) lipid-loading in macrophages; the smaller subspecies (S_f 100–400; S_f 60–100; S_f 20–60) did not. In contrast, the postprandial S_f 100–400 subfraction from subjects with abnormal fasting lipoprotein profiles (elevated VLDL and/or low HDL) caused up to a 10-fold increased macrophage lipid accumulation in a standard test for rapid, receptor-mediated lipid-loading, where postprandial TGRLP from normal subjects of the same relative size and lipid composition did not. The ability of the abnormal postprandial S_f 100 to 400 subfractions to cause lipid-loading changed with time postprandially, increasing up to 10-fold at 2 and 4 hr and returning to baseline by 8 hr. Consistent with the studies of others, which showed increased levels of plasma TG and chylomicrons and their remnants postprandially in HTG subjects (18,19), the levels of all TGRLP subclasses in hypertriglyceridemic subjects 2 to 6 hr postprandially were elevated six-to 10-fold relative to the levels of comparable subclasses in normal subjects. Because postprandial TGRLP from hypertriglyceridemic subjects are more active in causing macrophage lipid accumulation than normal TGRLP when compared on an equal particle basis, the TGRLP-induced atherogenicity of postprandial plasma is potentially far greater in hypertriglyceridemic subjects than in normal subjects due to increased numbers of particles with increased abilities to bind to both the LDL receptor and the modified VLDL receptor of macrophages.

These studies *in vitro* demonstrate abnormal cellular uptake of TGRLP, fasting and postprandial TGRLP, in subjects with certain hypertriglyceridemias. The abnormal TGRLP cause rapid cholesteryl ester and TG engorgement in macrophages and can convert endothelial cells into giant cells *in vitro*. We believe that these abnormal interactions are potentially atherogenic and may be causally related to the increased atherosclerosis associated with these disorders.

ACKNOWLEDGMENTS

This research was supported in part by grant HL43373 from the National Institutes of Health.

REFERENCES

1. Brown MS, Goldstein JL. Lipoprotein metabolism in the macrophage: implications for cholesterol deposition in atherosclerosis. *Ann Rev Biochem* 1983;52:223–261.
2. Ross R, Glomset JA. Atherosclerosis and the arterial smooth muscle cell. *Science* 1973;180:1332–1339.
3. Bradley WA, Hwang S-LC, Karlin JB, et al. Low-density lipoprotein receptor binding determinants switch from apolipoprotein E to apolipoprotein B during conversion of hypertriglyceridemic very-low-density lipoprotein to low-density lipoproteins. *J Biol Chem* 1984;259:14728–14735.
4. Gianturco SH, Gotto AM Jr, Jackson RL, et al. Control of 3-hydroxy-3-methylglytaryl-CoA reductase activity in cultured human fibroblasts by very low density lipoproteins of subjects with hypertriglyceridemia. *J Clin Invest* 1978;61:320–328.
5. Gianturco SH, Packard CJ, Shepherd J, et al. Abnormal suppression of 3-hydroxy-3-methylglutaryl-CoA reductase activity in cultured human fibroblasts by hypertriglyceridemic very low density lipoprotein subclasses. *Lipids* 1980;15:456–463.
6. Gianturco SH, Eskin SG, Navarro LT, Lahart CJ, Smith LC, Gotto AM Jr. Abnormal effects of hypertriacylglycerolemic very low-density lipoproteins on 3-hydroxy-3-methylglutaryl-CoA reductase activity and viability of cultured bovine aortic endothelial cells. *Biochim Biophys Acta* 1980;618:143–152.
7. Gianturco SH, Brown FB, Gotto AM Jr, Bradley WA. Receptor-mediated uptake of hypertriglyceridemic very low density lipoproteins by normal human fibroblasts. *J Lipid Res* 1982;23:984–993.
8. Gianturco SH, Bradley WA, Gotto AM Jr, Morrisett JD, Peavy DL. Hypertriglyceridemic very low density lipoproteins induce triglyceride synthesis and accumulation in mouse peritoneal macrophages. *J Clin Invest* 1982;70:168–178.
9. Gianturco SH, Gotto AM Jr, Hwang S-LC, et al. Apolipoprotein E mediates uptake of S_f 100–400 hypertriglyceridemic very low density lipoproteins by the low density lipoprotein receptor pathway in normal human fibroblasts. *J Biol Chem* 1983;258:4526–4533

10. Gianturco SH, Brown SA, Via DP, Bradley WA. The β-VLDL receptor pathway of murine P388D$_1$ macrophages. *J Lipid Res* 1986;27:412–420.
11. Gianturco SH, Lin AH-Y, Hwang S-LC, et al. Distinct murine macrophage receptor pathway for human triglyceride-rich lipoproteins. *J Clin Invest* 1988;82;1633–1643.
12. Gianturco SH, Lin AH-Y, Ramprasad MP, Song R, Bradley WA. Monocyte-macrophage receptor pathway for abnormal triglyceride-rich lipoproteins. In: Gotto AM Jr, Smith LC, eds. *Drugs affecting lipid metabolism X.* Amsterdam:Elsevier, 1990:261–264.
13. Frederickson DS, Goldstein JL, Brown MS. The familial hyperlipoproteinemias. In: Stanbury JG, Wyngaarden MF, Fredrickson DS, eds. *The metabolic basis of inherited diseases.* 4th ed. New York: McGraw-Hill, 1978;604–655.
14. Shen BW, Scanu AM, Kézdy FJ. Structure of human serum lipoproteins inferred from compositional analysis. *Proc Natl Acad Sci USA* 1977;74:837–841.
15. Packard CJ, Munro A, Lorimer AR, Gotto AM, Shepherd J. Metabolism of apolipoprotein B in large triglyceride-rich very low density lipoproteins of normal and hypertriglyceridemic subjects. *J Clin Invest* 1984;74:2178–2192.
16. Eisenberg S, Friedman G, Vogel T. Enhanced metabolism of normolipidemic human plasma very low density lipoprotein in cultured cells by exogenous apolipoprotein E-3. *Arteriosclerosis* 1988;8:480–487.
17. Zilversmit DB. Atherogenesis: a postprandial phenomenon. *Circulation* 1979;60:473–485.
18. Weintraub MS, Eisenberg S, Breslow JL. Different patterns of postprandial lipoprotein metabolism in normal, type IIa, type III, and type IV hyperlipoproteinemic individuals. *J Clin Invest* 1987;79:1110–1119.
19. Patsch JR, Karlin JB, Scott LW, Smith LC, Gotto AM Jr. Inverse relationship between blood levels of high density lipoprotein subfraction 2 and magnitude of postprandial lipemia. *Proc Natl Acad Sci USA* 1983;80:1449–1453.

Atherosclerosis Reviews, Volume 22,
edited by A. M. Gotto, Jr. and R. Paoletti.
Raven Press, Ltd., New York © 1991.

Role of Hypertriglyceridemia in Abnormal High-Density Lipoprotein ApoA-I Metabolism

Henry N. Ginsberg, Colleen Ngai, and
Rajasekhar Ramakrishnan

*Department of Medicine, College of Physicians and Surgeons,
Columbia University, New York, New York 10032*

Reduced plasma concentrations of high-density lipoprotein (HDL) cholesterol are commonly associated with high plasma levels of very-low-density lipoprotein (VLDL) triglycerides (TG). Two possible mechanisms have been suggested as the basis of this relationship. First, it has been suggested that defective lipolysis of TG-rich lipoproteins (VLDL or chylomicrons) results in diminished generation of surface components such as free cholesterol, phospholipids, and the C-apolipoproteins that could be utilized for HDL production in plasma. This hypothesis is supported both by data demonstrating transfer of these components from TG-rich lipoproteins (TGRLP) to HDL and the strong, inverse relationship between either plasma or adipose tissue lipoprotein lipase (LPL) activity and HDL cholesterol levels in plasma.

Second, accelerated exchange of HDL core cholesteryl ester for VLDL and/or chylomicron core TG, via the plasma mediator, cholesteryl ester transfer protein (CETP), has been proposed as the basis for low plasma HDL cholesterol concentrations in hypertriglyceridemia. *In vitro* studies by several investigators have demonstrated accelerated transfer of HDL cholesteryl ester in the presence of increased quantities of acceptor TGRLP. These studies have been supported by measurements of cholesteryl ester mass transfer during the postprandial period in normal and hyperlipidemic subjects. It has also been suggested that diabetic subjects have increased transfer of HDL cholesteryl ester to VLDL. The importance of CETP in the regulation of plasma HDL cholesterol concentration has received further support from the recent identification and study of patients with absence of CETP and extreme elevations of plasma HDL cholesterol concentrations.

Several issues related to the pathophysiologic basis of low HDL levels remain unanswered. One major issue is the relationship between hypertriglyceridemia and reduced plasma HDL cholesterol levels. For example, it has been demonstrated that reduction in plasma VLDL TG, achieved either by weight loss or physical activity, rarely raise an individual's HDL cholesterol concentrations to normal (1,2). Indeed, individuals who start with HDL cholesterol levels below 30 mg/dl rarely raise their levels above 35 mg/dl, even when plasma TG levels are dramatically reduced. This limitation in increasing HDL cholesterol levels even extends to pharmacotherapy. Therefore, it is not startling that some patients actually present with low plasma HDL cholesterol levels and normal plasma TG concentrations (3). Clearly, individuals with low HDL cholesterol and normal plasma TG levels do not reflect the typical relationship between VLDL TG and HDL cholesterol seen in the general population. Taken together, these findings suggest that the link between hypertriglyceridemia and low HDL cholesterol concentrations may be indirect, via another abnormality in lipid metabolism.

Previous studies have found that the rates of production of apolipoprotein B (apoB) in both VLDL and low-density lipoprotein (LDL) are elevated in hypertriglyceridemic subjects (4). ApoB production is also elevated in subjects with combined hyperlipidemia (CHL) who may or may not have hypertriglyceridemia (5–7). Hence, one possible link between the variable presence of elevated VLDL TG levels in individuals with low HDL cholesterol concentrations could be abnormalities in apoB metabolism. Such a defect would very likely increase the probability, but not absolutely predetermine, that an individual would be hypertriglyceridemic. On the other hand, it remains unclear how increased apoB production could be related to low HDL cholesterol levels in the absence of absolute hypertriglyceridemia.

The finding that apoA-I, the major structural protein in HDL, is also reduced in subjects with low HDL cholesterol levels adds another level of complexity to this issue that requires explanation. Although the underlying mechanism for reduced apoA-I levels in these individuals is unknown, we do know that increased HDL apoA-I fractional catabolic rates (FCR) can be demonstrated in subjects with low HDL cholesterol levels and hypertriglyceridemia (8–10). Could this alteration in HDL apoA-I metabolism be linked to abnormalities in VLDL and LDL apoB metabolism? To address this issue, we studied HDL apoA-I FCR and LDL apoB metabolism in subjects with low HDL cholesterol and normal plasma concentrations of VLDL TG and LDL cholesterol. The results have been compared to data obtained in previous studies of LDL and HDL metabolism in subjects with normal TG and normal HDL cholesterol levels and in subjects with hypertriglyceridemia and low HDL cholesterol concentrations.

Our results demonstrate that subjects with reduced plasma concentrations of HDL cholesterol and normal plasma TG levels have several metabolic characteristics in common with their hypertriglyceridemic counterparts. For example, compared to subjects with normal HDL cholesterol levels, subjects with low HDL cholesterol (<35 mg/dl) have about a 30% increase in HDL apoA-I FCR regardless of their plasma TG levels. Of note in this regard was the finding that the subjects with normal plasma TG and low HDL cholesterol levels had abnormal HDL cholesterol:TG ratios. Thus, while the ratio was about 6:1 in normal controls, it was about 4:1 in the normal TG/low HDL cholesterol group. The ratio was even lower—2:1—in the hypertriglyceridemic subjects. The basis of abnormal cholesterol:TG ratios in subjects with normal plasma TG levels is unclear, but this abnormality might play a role in their HDL apoA-I FCR. Indeed, the fractional catabolic rates for HDL apoA-I were inversely correlated with the cholesterol:TG ratio in HDL ($r = -0.80$).

Subjects with reduced plasma HDL cholesterol levels also were found to have elevated rates of LDL apoB flux in plasma whether or not they were hypertriglyceridemic. Both the hypertriglyceridemic and the normotriglyceridemic individuals with low HDL cholesterol had production rates of LDL apoB that were 50% greater than the production rates in the normal subjects. Hence, a second defect common to both groups with low HDL cholesterol, this time involving the metabolism of the apoB-containing lipoproteins, was demonstrated to be independent of plasma TG levels. These results, together with previous data from our laboratory and from other investigators demonstrating oversecretion of apoB-containing lipoproteins into plasma in subjects with combined hyperlipidemia, suggest that our two groups with low HDL cholesterol may have had this latter lipid phenotype as their underlying metabolic abnormality. The hypertriglyceridemia in one of the groups may be the result of slightly greater adiposity, less physical activity, or genetic predispositions that add to an underlying pathophysiology of overproduction of apoB-containing lipoproteins. In this light, it is interesting to note that some of the normal TG patients in this group either had first-degree relatives with hypertriglyceridemia or had an occasional hypertriglyceridemic value themselves some time prior to the study.

How might overproduction of apoB-containing lipoproteins relate to reduced HDL cholesterol levels and increased apoA-I fractional catabolism? Both mechanisms proposed as bases for the inverse relationship between plasma TG levels and HDL cholesterol concentrations could, even in the absence of significant hypertriglyceridemia, result in altered HDL composition. Thus, increased secretion of nascent VLDL might trap surface components such as C-apolipoproteins, phospholipids, and free cholesterol that are generated by LPL-lipolysis of circulating VLDL TG, within the VLDL density range. As a consequence of inadequate transfer of these surface components from VLDL to HDL, apoA-I fractional catabolism could increase. Alternatively, even in the absence of increased plasma VLDL TG levels, increased numbers of VLDL (or IDL) particles might still serve as substrate for CETP-mediated exchange of TG for HDL cholesteryl ester. An additional possibility is the accumulation of a particular VLDL or IDL subclass (in both hypertriglyceridemic and normal TG-high apoB subjects) that is a unique substrate for CETP-mediated transfer. In either case, HDL lipid-core composition would be altered, and this might, in turn, lead to accelerated apoA-I FCR.

How might these findings relate to low HDL cholesterol levels in diabetics, particularly in patients with type II diabetes mellitus? Certainly, if hypertriglyceridemia is present, the above-described mechanisms would alter HDL lipid/apolipoprotein composition and accelerate apoA-I FCR. A more significant factor, we believe, is the overproduction of apoB in VLDL and LDL that is common in type II diabetes mellitus (11,12). ApoB production, possibly driven by increased free fatty acid flux to the liver, by altered carbohydrate metabolism, or by insulin itself could be the basis of abnormal HDL metabolism in type II diabetics (13). Hence, therapeutic regimens aimed at reducing free fatty acid flux and normalizing glucose metabolism should increase plasma HDL cholesterol concentrations and normalize HDL apoA-I metabolism in these patients.

REFERENCES

1. Witzum JL, Dillingham MA, Giese W, et al. Normalization of triglycerides in type IV hyperlipoproteinemia fails to correct low levels of high density lipoprotein cholesterol. *N Engl J Med* 1980;303:907–914.
2. Nicoll A, Miller NE, Lewis B. High density lipoprotein metabolism. *Adv Lipid Res* 1980;17:53–105.
3. Ordovas JM, Schaefer EJ, Salem D, et al. Apolipoprotein A-I gene polymorphism associated with premature coronary artery disease and familial hypoalphalipoproteinemia. *N Engl J Med* 1986;314:671–677.
4. Ginsberg HN, Le N-A, Gibson JC. Regulation of production and catabolism of plasma low density lipoproteins in hypertriglyceridemic subjects. The effects of weight loss. *J Clin Invest* 1985;75:614–623.
5. Teng B, Sniderman AD, Soutar, AK, Thompson GR. Metabolic basis of hyperapobetalipoproteinemia: turnover of apolipoprotein B in low density lipoprotein and its precursors and subfractions compared with normal and familial hypercholesterolemia. *J Clin Invest* 1986;77:663–672.
6. Kissebah AH, Alfarsi S, Adamo PW. Integrated regulation of very low density lipoprotein triglyceride and apolipoprotein-B kinetics in man: normolipidemic subjects, familial hypertriglyceridemia and familial combined hyperlipidemia. *Metabolism* 1981;30:856–868.
7. Arad Y, Ramakrishnan R, Ginsberg HN. Lovastatin therapy reduces low density lipoprotein apoB levels in subjects with combined hyperlipidemia by reducing the production of apoB-containing lipoproteins: implications for the pathophysiology of apoB production. *J Lipid Res* 1990;31:567–582.
8. Fidge N, Nestel P, Ishikawa T, et al. Turnover of apoproteins A-I and A-II of high density lipoprotein and the relationship to other lipoproteins in normal and hyperlipidemic individuals. *Metabolism* 1980;29:643–653.
9. Saku K, Garside PS, Hynd BA, et al. Apolipoprotein AI and AII metabolism in patients with primary high density lipoprotein deficiency associated with familial hypertriglyceridemia. *Metabolism* 1985;34:754–764.
10. Le N-A, Ginsberg HN. Heterogeneity of apolipoprotein A-I turnover in subjects with reduced concentrations of plasma high density lipoprotein cholesterol. *Metabolism* 1988;37:614–617.
11. Kissebah AH, Alfarsi S, Evans DJ, Adams PW. Integrated regulation of very low density

lipoprotein triglyceride and apolipoprotein-B kinetics in non–insulin-dependent diabetes mellitus. *Diabetes* 1982;31:217–225.

12. Ginsberg HN. Very low density lipoprotein metabolism in diabetes mellitus. *Diabetes Metab Rev* 1987;3:571–589.

13. Chen Y-DI, Jeng C-Y, Reaven GM. HDL metabolism in diabetes. *Diabetes Metab Rev* 1987;3:653–668.

Atherosclerosis Reviews, Volume 22,
edited by A. M. Gotto, Jr. and R. Paoletti.
Raven Press, Ltd., New York © 1991.

Lipoprotein Lipase

Sites of Synthesis and Sites of Action

Thomas Olivecrona, Gunilla Bengtsson-Olivecrona, *Tova
Chajek-Shaul, †Yvon Carpentier, ‡Richard Deckelbaum,
Magnus Hultin, Jonas Peterson, §Josef Patsch, and
‖Senén Vilaró

*Departments of Medical Biochemistry and Biophysics, University of Umeå, S-901
87 Sweden; *Medicine I, Hadassah University Hospital, Il-91 120 Jerusalem,
Israel; †Clinical Nutrition, Free University of Brussels, B-1000 Brussels, Belgium,
‡Pediatrics, Columbia University, New York, New York 10032; §Medizinische
Universitätsklinik, A-6020 Innsbruck, Austria; and ‖Cell Biology,
University of Barcelona, E-08028 Barcelona, Spain*

There are two major pathways by which the lipids from chylomicra and VLDL are delivered to tissue cells: lipoprotein lipase (LPL)-catalyzed hydrolysis of triglycerides, and receptor-mediated endocytosis of cholesterol-rich remnant lipoproteins (Fig. 1). Both pathways are believed to be regulated locally, but the conditions for regulation are different for the two. The receptors are made within the cells that engage the lipoproteins, and the lipids are brought into these cells. LPL, on the other hand, is made within lipid-metabolizing parenchymal cells, but it is delivered to and acts at the luminal side of the vascular endothelium. There is evidence for a correlation between local production of LPL and the uptake of fatty acids from lipoprotein triglycerides (TG) in the tissue. For instance, Scow and Chernick have shown a strong relation between the uptake of chylomicron lipids by the lactating mammary gland and the LPL activity in the gland (1). Other authors have investigated the correlation between lipid uptake and LPL activity in adipose tissue (2).

LPL is thought to be attached to endothelial cells via interaction with heparan sulfate (Fig. 2). There must be continuous dissociation and reassociation of the lipase as well as potential for transport to other parts of the vascular mesh. The products of lipase action, free fatty acids (FFA) and monoglycerides, are available for local uptake, but they can also recirculate in blood. We wish to consider the importance of these transport processes for the metabolism of triglyceride-rich lipoproteins (TGRLP).

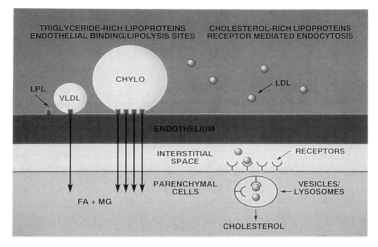

FIG. 1. The two major mechanisms for delivery of lipoprotein lipids to cells.

Recent studies have found LPL mRNA in many tissues, demonstrating widespread synthesis of the enzyme (3,4). To further localize the sites of lipase production, we used *in situ* hybridization of LPL mRNA combined with immunolocalization of LPL protein (5,6). Our findings corroborated several previous studies, showing strong reaction over the dominant parenchymal cells in adipose tissue and muscles, i.e., adipocytes/preadipocytes and myocytes. In other tissues, only certain cells gave positive reaction for LPL. In some tissues, e.g., lungs—these cells were macrophages. In other tissues, LPL was made in specialized cells, e.g., neuronal cells in the hip-

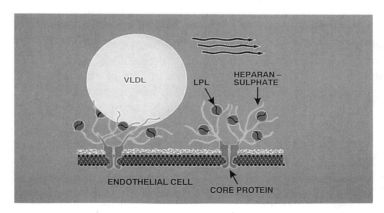

FIG. 2. Illustration of how TG-rich lipoproteins may interact with LPL at the vascular endothelium.

pocampus and some other parts of the nervous system; in addition, some of the hormone produced cells in adrenals and ovaries (7,8).

There is a low but definite LPL activity in basal plasma (9,10). This activity is <1% of the activity obtained after heparin injection, which is thought to give a measure of the amount of LPL available at endothelial sites. The reported dissociation constants for binding of LPL to endothelial cells are 0.14 μM or more (11). Taken together, these figures indicate that binding-site occupancy must be low. This finding would be expected because heparan sulfate proteoglycans are ubiquitous components of endothelial cells throughout the body.

LPL released into the circulating blood from tissues synthesizing the enzyme should be able to bind to endothelial sites in other tissues. The hypothesis that vascular endothelium can bind large amounts of LPL was put to a direct test by perfusing rat hearts with exogenous ^{125}I-labeled LPL (12). Binding was proportional to the concentration of perfused lipase up to 50 nM, the highest concentration studied. The bound lipase behaved similarly to endogenous LPL in that it retained its catalytic activity, could hydrolyze perfused TG, and was rapidly released back to the medium by heparin. During chase perfusion, the labeled LPL slowly returned to the medium at a rate of ~2.5%/min; this was similar to the rate at which endogenous LPL was released. There was no evidence for degradation of the exogenous lipase. These results indicate that endothelial LPL exchanges with lipase in blood and that a major route for turnover is transport in blood, with net uptake and degradation in the liver.

Studies where labeled LPL was injected to intact rats showed binding of lipase in all tissues (unpublished data). Studies using immunofluorescence showed reaction at endothelial surfaces of all vessels in virtually all tissues (5,6). At some sites, the endothelial LPL could have come from nearby parenchymal cells that synthesize the lipase, but the enzyme found in other vessels must have been carried by the bloodstream. For instance, there was intense immunoreaction for LPL in the aorta, but only a few cells in the deeper layers of the vessel wall reacted for LPL protein or LPL mRNA. We also noted a strong immunoreaction for LPL in the glomeruli of the kidney, but there was no evidence for local synthesis.

These observations suggest that a substantial amount of LPL is transported in blood. The concentration of LPL in blood has been found to differ in various metabolic situations. For instance, compared to the basal state, LPL activity in blood rises during fasting (10), after adrenergic stimulation (9), and after treatment with tumor necrosis factor (14). The most marked increase, however, occurs postprandially. Postprandial changes were studied in a group of 50 middle-aged men with a wide range of lipid and lipoprotein concentrations (J. Patsch and T. Olivecrona, unpublished data). Plasma LPL activity increased after a peronal fat load meal in all but one of the subjects. All of the subjects who registered large rises of plasma TG also had large rises of plasma LPL. However, equally large increases of LPL activity were seen in several of the subjects who registered small or moderate increases in plasma TG. Elevated TG levels in basal plasma were not associated with increased plasma LPL activity. Hence, the elevation of plasma LPL was not directly related to the concentration of TG in plasma, but it was associated with the postprandial transport of TG.

In another study of this phenomenon, Peterson et al. created an experimental overloading of the TG clearing system by infusing Intralipid at a high rate to fasting volunteers (15). The dose—0.3 g/kg body weight per hour—approximated the potential rate of endothelial LPL hydrolysis but far exceeded the subjects' immediate energy needs. The infusion caused a progressive rise of plasma TG in all the subjects. It also caused increases of plasma free fatty acids (FFA), but the increases varied among the individuals. Plasma LPL activity also rose. This increase was correlated to FFA but not to TG, both with respect to the levels reached and to the time course. In ongoing studies, similar results have been obtained in rats infused with lipid emulsions and in humans after oral fat loads.

Earlier *in vitro* studies (15) have shown that LPL binds fatty acids and that the resulting complexes have much-reduced affinities for lipid/water interfaces, for apolipoprotein C-II, and for heparin-like polysaccharides. Moreover, Saxena et al. recently showed that physiologic concentrations of fatty acids dissociate LPL from cultured endothelial cells (16). This finding suggests the following sequence of events: Fatty acids can be released by LPL at endothelial sites more rapidly than the underlying tissue is capable of transporting or metabolizing them. The result is spillage of fatty acids into the blood and the formation of LPL–fatty acid complexes. This leads to dissociation of LPL from endothelial heparan sulfate, which in turn leads to a cessation of ongoing hydrolysis. By implication, there must be situations in which LPL is present in excess, and the real limitation for hydrolysis of lipoprotein TG is transport and metabolism of fatty acids by the underlying tissue.

In conclusion, lipid delivery by LPL-catalyzed hydrolysis is less localized than delivery of lipids by receptor-mediated uptake of remnant lipoproteins. In situations with high plasma TG and limited capacity for fatty acid utilization in some tissues, product control of LPL action rather than total LPL availability may govern the reaction, and there may be extensive transport in blood of both the enzyme itself and the fatty acids resulting from TG hydrolysis.

ACKNOWLEDGMENTS

This study was supported by grants from the Swedish Medical Research Council (B31-727) and from the Swedish Margarine Industry Fund for research in nutrition to T.O. and G.B.-O.; grant 9.4501.88 from Fonds Belgé de la Recherche Scientifique Medicale to Y.A.C.; grant P50 21006 from the National Institutes of Health to R.J.D.; and grants from Comisión Asesora de Investigatión y Ciencia and the Generalitat de Catalunya (AR87, CIRIT) to S.V.

REFERENCES

1. Scow RO, Chernick SC. Role of lipoprotein lipase during lactation. In: Borensztajn J, ed. *Lipoprotein lipase*. Chicago: Evener, 1987;149–185.
2. Cryer A, Riley SE, Williams ER, Robinson DS. Effect of nutritional status on rat adipose tissue, muscle and post-heparin plasma clearing factor lipase activities: their relationship to triglyceride fatty acid uptake by fat-cells and to plasma insulin concentrations. *Clin Sci Mol Med* 1976;50:213–221.
3. Semenkovich CF, Chen S-H, Wims M, Luo C-C, Li W-H, Chan L. Lipoprotein lipase and hepatic lipase mRNA tissue specific expression, developmental regulation, and evolution. *J Lipid Res* 1989;30:423–431.
4. Kirchgessner TG, LeBoeuf RC, Langner CA, et al. Genetic and developmental regulation of the lipoprotein lipase gene: loci both distal and proximal to the lipoprotein lipase structural gene control enzyme expression. *J Biol Chem* 1989;264:1473–1482.
5. Camps L, Reina M, Llobera M, Vilaró S, Olivecrona T. Lipoprotein lipase: cellular origin and functional distribution. *Am J Physiol* 1990;258:C673–C681.
6. Camps L, Reina M, Llobera M, Olivecrona T, Vilaró S. Lipoprotein lipase in lungs, spleen and liver: synthesis and distribution. *J Lipid Res* (in press).
7. Vilaró S, Camps L, Reina M, Perez-Clausell J, Llobera M, Olivecrona T. Localization of lipoprotein lipase to discrete areas of the guinea pig brain. *Brain Res* 1990;506:249–253.
8. Camps L, Gåfvels M, Reina M, Wallin C, Vilaró S, Olivecrona T. Expression of lipoprotein lipase in ovaries of the guinea pig. *Biol Reprod* (in press).
9. Knobler H, Chajek-Shaul T, Stein O, Etienne J, Stein Y. Modulation of lipoprotein lipase in the intact rat by cholera toxin—an irreversible agonist of cyclic AMP. *Biochim Biophys Acta* 1984;795:363–371.
10. Peterson J, Olivecrona T, Bengtsson-Olivecrona G. Distribution of lipoprotein lipase and hepatic lipase between plasma and tissues: effect of hypertriglyceridemia. *Biochim Biophys Acta* 1985;837:262–270.
11. Shimada K, Gill PJ, Silbert JE, Douglas WHJ, Fanburg BL. Involvement of cell surface heparan sulfate in the binding of lipoprotein lipase to cultured bovine endothelial cells. *J Clin Invest* 1981;68:995–1002.
12. Chajek-Shaul T, Bengtsson-Olivecrona G, Peterson J, Olivecrona T. Metabolic fate of rat heart endothelial lipoprotein lipase. *Am J Physiol* 1988;255:E247–E254.
13. Chajek-Shaul T, Friedman G, Stein O, Shiloni E, Etienne J. Mechanism of the hypertriglyceridemia induced by tumor necrosis factor administration to rats. *Biochem Biophys Acta* 1989;1001:316–324.
14. Semb H, Peterson J, Tavernier J, Olivecrona T. Multiple effect of tumor necrosis factor on lipoprotein lipase in vivo. *J Biol Chem* 1987;262:8390–8394.
15. Peterson J, Bihain BE, Bengtsson-Olivecrona G, Deckelbaum RJ, Carpentier YA, Olivecrona T. Fatty acid control of lipoprotein lipase: a link between energy metabolism and lipid transport. *Proc Natl Acad Sci USA* 1990;87:909–913.
16. Saxena U, Witte LD, Goldberg IJ. Release of endothelial cell lipoprotein lipase by plasma lipoproteins and free fatty acids. *J Biol Chem* 1989;264:4349–4355.

Atherosclerosis Reviews, Volume 22,
edited by A. M. Gotto, Jr. and R. Paoletti.
Raven Press, Ltd., New York © 1991.

Insulin Regulation of Triglyceride Metabolism

George Steiner

*Division of Endocrinology and Metabolism, Toronto General Hospital,
Ontario, Canada M5G 2C4*

The most frequent form of hyperlipidemia in the diabetic is hypertriglyceridemia (1,2). For the small minority of the diabetic population who are severely out of control, lipoprotein lipase (LPL) activity is greatly reduced, with a consequent impairment in the ability to remove chylomicrons. However, most diabetics with hypertriglyceridemia show an increase in the level of smaller-sized very-low-density lipoproteins (VLDL) and intermediate-density lipoproteins (IDL) (3; unpublished observations).

Most diabetics are hyperinsulinemic. If profound insulin deficiency were to continue, the patient would succumb to diabetic ketoacidosis; therefore, this condition is not seen in the general diabetic population. Patients with non–insulin-dependent diabetes (NIDDM) generally have insulin resistance. In these cases, the pancreas attempts to compensate by secreting more insulin. As a result, hyperinsulinemia will occur at least in the hepatic portal circulation. When the pancreas cannot secrete sufficient insulin to achieve metabolic control, insulin must be administered by a peripheral route. In order to deliver the appropriate insulin concentration into the hepatic circulation, hyperinsulinemia is once again produced. This time it is primarily peripheral.

Therefore, when our laboratory set out to study lipoprotein metabolism in diabetes with an aim to understanding some of the factors involved in the high rate of atherosclerosis in the diabetic, we began by examining the effect of chronic hyperinsulinemia on the metabolism of VLDL-triglyceride (TG).

CHRONIC ENDOGENOUS HYPERINSULINEMIA IN HUMANS

In humans, chronic endogenous (i.e., pancreatic) hyperinsulinemia occurs most commonly in connection with obesity. Therefore, we studied obese individuals in order to examine the effects of chronic changes in endogenous insulin levels on the metabolism of VLDL TG (4). All subjects underwent a 4-week total fast as part of a weight-loss program. VLDL TG kinetics were studied before the fast, at its conclusion, and after a period of hypocaloric refeeding. No correlation was found either with any changes in weight or with any other anthropometric index. However, the rate of TG production correlated positively with serum levels of insulin. Similar correlations have also been found between the rate of TG production and serum levels of insulin in individuals receiving glucocorticoid therapy (5). Because both of these models had, of course, many other variables, we deemed it necessary to turn to a more controllable *in vivo* model to pursue our investigation.

THE CHRONICALLY HYPERINSULINEMIC RAT

The model for these studies was originally described by Kobayashi and Olefsky (6). Rats were treated with insulin in doses up to 6 U per rat per day for a period of 2 weeks. In order to prevent profound hypoglycemia, a 10% sugar solution was substituted for the rats' drinking water. A control group was given a similar 10% sugar solution to drink but not treated with insulin. Since the controls also developed hyperinsulinemia that derived from the pancreas, they provided a model of endogenous hyperinsulinemia, whereas the insulin-treated group provided a model of exogenous hyperinsulinemia.

In some cases, the insulin was given subcutaneously (peripheral route), while in others it was given intraperitoneally (portal route). Both types of insulin delivery resulted in the same increase in portal venous insulin concentration. However, rats receiving the insulin subcutaneously had a much higher peripheral venous insulin concentration than those receiving insulin intraperitoneally (7). The increase reflected the transhepatic extraction of the portally delivered insulin.

The hyperinsulinemic rats showed an increase in rate of VLDL TG production (7–10). This increase was the same in both the exogenous and endogenous groups. In rats receiving insulin peripherally, the plasma concentration of TG fell, reflecting an increase in the activity of lipoprotein lipase (LPL), which permitted TG to be removed faster than it was being produced. In rats receiving insulin via the portal vein, TG removal was somewhat less accelerated, so TG concentration rose (7).

Hyperinsulinemia also led to a reduction in the plasma concentration of free fatty acids (FFA) (9). Thus, a greater proportion of the FA of the TG had to be derived from a source other than plasma FFA. It was noteworthy that in rats receiving fructose rather than glucose as the sugar in their drinking solution, insulin caused a greater increase in TG synthesis. This may have been due to the fact that an oral load of fructose is removed primarily by the liver, whereas most oral glucose is removed by extrahepatic tissues. Thus, fructose may provide a better substrate for the production of FA in the TG.

CONTROVERSY ARISING FROM HEPATOCYTE STUDIES

Several laboratories have studied the effects of adding insulin to the medium in which hepatocytes are cultured (11–17). They have generally observed that exposure to insulin for periods in the range of 16 to 24 hr results in a decrease in the amounts of both VLDL apoB and TG appearing in the medium even when there is an increase in the amounts of each in the cells. At first glance, these findings appear to conflict with the *in vivo* data. Some studies have shown that in the presence of glucorticoids, insulin may have little effect or may even be stimulatory rather than inhibitory (15,16). This would suggest that *in vivo*, the chronically hyperinsulinemic state reflects the interaction of several hormones. Other investigators have suggested that hepatocytes incubated for longer with insulin may develop a resistance to insulin, and the secretion of VLDL may increase (17). Thus, duration of exposure to insulin would be a significant factor in our understanding of the chronically hyperinsulinemic state. We therefore undertook to examine the immediate effects of insulin on the production of VLDL.

IMMEDIATE EFFECTS OF INSULIN ON VLDL TG PRODUCTION IN HUMANS

In our studies of human subjects, the rate of VLDL TG production was estimated qualitatively by following the slope of the curve describing the decline of TG specific activity after an injection of [^{3}H]glycerol (17). We monitored the decline for a 6-hr basal period. Thereafter, the volunteer was started on a 6-hr euglycemic hyperinsulinemic clamp. The VLDL pool size decreased for the first 3 hr, then reached a new, lower plateau in the final 3 hr. Next, the slope of the specific activity curve during the final 3 hr was compared to that recorded in the basal 6 hr. Even if there had been no increase in the rate of VLDL TG production, the reduction in the pool size itself would have resulted in an increased fractional turnover rate and therefore a steeper slope. It was possible to estimate how much steeper this slope would have been. In only one of seven individuals was the slope actually steeper. Thus, we concluded that during short-term exposure to exogenous insulin, the rate of VLDL TG production does not increase. At first glance, this hypothesis appears to be consistent with the observations in the studies of cultured rat hepatocytes.

IMMEDIATE EFFECTS OF INSULIN ON VLDL TG PRODUCTION IN RATS

The studies using human volunteers are also consistent with the data of Alcindor et al., whose work showed that the rate of VLDL TG production in rats decreases immediately after an injection of insulin (18). We have repeated those experiments, with the same results (unpublished observations). In addition, we found that the plasma concentration of FFA declined following an injection of insulin. This finding corroborates our earlier observations in humans (17). We then tried to determine whether a reduction in one of the substrates for VLDL-TG would cause a reduction in the rate of VLDL TG production in rats. For this experiment, we infused FFA to prevent the fall of plasma FFA, measured VLDL TG production during a basal period, injected insulin, and remeasured the production of VLDL TG (unpublished observations). Results showed that when the FFA did not decline, the rate of VLDL TG production actually increased. Thus, if the supply of FFA is not reduced, the immediate response to insulin *in vivo* is an increase in the rate of VLDL TG production.

STUDIES WITH PERFUSED RAT LIVERS

To examine the effects of insulin more directly, we turned to an *in vitro* system. For this investigation, we chose to use the isolated perfused liver, because it is a system that is closer to human physiology than isolated hepatocytes. Because the rate of oxygen supply, as influenced by both the hematocrit of the perfusate and the rate of perfusion, can influence the metabolic behavior of the liver (19,20), we undertook perfusions in which the hematocrit was 37% and the rate of perfusion was 16 ml/min.

Our initial studies compared the livers of normal rats to those of rats made hyperinsulinemic over a 2-week period by either exogenous insulin administration or by stimulating the release of endogenous insulin by substituting 10% glucose for drinking water. Livers from both of the hyperinsulinemic groups took up FFA from the perfusate at the same rate as normal livers. However, the livers from both groups of hyperinsulinemic rats produced more VLDL TG than livers from normal rats. Thus, the effects of the chronically hyperinsulinemic state on VLDL TG production by the isolated livers was identical to that observed in the whole animal. This finding indicates that VLDL TG production in the chronically hyperinsulinemic state is a function of the liver rather than a metabolic process in some other tissue.

Next, we examined the effects of adding insulin to the medium of isolated perfused normal livers. The insulin had no effect on the rate of FFA uptake; it suppressed glucose production, and it increased the rate of VLDL TG production (unpublished observations). Thus, as in the *in vivo* studies, when FFA remained available, the immediate response of the liver to insulin was to increase the production of VLDL TG.

The reasons for the differences between the two *in vitro* systems—the perfused livers and the isolated hepatocytes—have not yet been elucidated. These differences include (a) the maintenance of the architectural integrity of the liver in the perfused organ system, (b) the presence of more than one cell type in the whole organ, (c) differences in the delivery of substrates and O_2 between the circulation and the incubation medium, (d) differences between the composition of the perfusate and the incubation medium, to name just a few. It is also possible that the isolated perfused liver is still under the influence of its immediately antecedent hormonal and substrate environment.

MODULATORS OF INSULIN'S EFFECT ON VLDL TG PRODUCTION *IN VIVO*

There are many factors that can influence the *in vivo* effects of insulin on VLDL TG production. Some of these factors relate to insulin itself—e.g., its concentration, the route and timing of its delivery, and the body's sensitivity to insulin. It is important to recognize that an individual's sensitivity and resistance may differ from one organ to another and from one metabolic pathway to another. The effects of insulin on VLDL TG production can also be influenced by the availability and the nature of the substrates for TG fatty acid synthesis. Factors include the type of the carbohydrate consumed (i.e., fructose versus glucose) and the availability of FFA in the circulation. The levels of other hormones, such as glucagon, epinephrine, and the glucocorticoids, can also modulate insulin's action. The following metabolic pathways in the liver, which are ultimately involved in the production of VLDL, can also be influenced by insulin: (a) the rate of hepatic lipogenesis, (b) the rate of FA esterification versus oxidation, (c) the rate of apoB production, and (d) the assembly and secretion of the final VLDL product. Clearly, the effect of insulin on the production of VLDL *in vivo* is determined by the balance among all of these factors.

REFERENCES

1. Zimmerman BR, Palumbo PJ, O'Fallon WA, et al. A prospective study of peripheral arterial occlusive disease in diabetics, III. Initial lipid and lipoprotein findings. *Mayo Clin Proc* 1981;56:223–242.
2. Barrett-Connor E, Grundy SM, Holdbrook MJ. Plasma lipids and diabetes mellitus in an adult community. *Am J Epidemiol* 1982;115:657–663.
3. Poapst M, Reardon M, Steiner G. Relative contribution of triglyceride-rich lipoprotein particle size and number to plasma triglyceride concentration. *Arteriosclerosis* 1985;5:381–390.
4. Streja DA, Marliss EB, Steiner G. The effect of prolonged fasting on plasma triglyceride kinetics in man. *Metabolism* 1976;26:505–516.
5. Cattran DC, Steiner G, Wilson DR, et al. Hyperlipidemia after renal transplantation: natural history and pathology. *Ann Intern Med* 1979;91:554–559.
6. Kobayashi M, Olefsky JM. Effect of experimental hyperinsulinemia on insulin binding and glucose transport in isolated rat hepatocytes. *Am J Physiol* 1978;235:E53–E62.
7. Kazumi T, Vranic M, Bar-On H, Steiner G. Portal v peripheral hyperinsulinemia and very low density lipoprotein triglyceride kinetics. *Metabolism* 1986;35:1024–1028.

8. Kazumi T, Vranic M, Steiner G. Triglyceride kinetics: effects of dietary glucose, sucrose or fructose alone or with hyperinsulinemia. *Am J Physiol* 1986;250:E325–E330.

9. Steiner G, Haynes FJ, Yoshino G, Vranic M. Hyperinsulinemia and in vivo very-low-density lipoprotein-triglyceride kinetics. *Am J Physiol* 1984;246:E187–E192.

10. Kazumi T, Vranic M, Steiner G. Changes in VLDL particle size and production in response to sucrose feeding and hyperinsulinemia. *Endocrinology* 1985;117:1145–1150.

11. Patsch W, Franz S, Schonfeld G. Role of insulin in lipoprotein secretion by cultured rat hepatocytes. *J Clin Invest* 1983;71:1161–1174.

12. Durrington PN, Newton RS, Weinstein DB, et al. The effect of insulin and glucose on very low density lipoprotein triglyceride secretion by cultured rat hepatocytes. *J Clin Invest* 1982;70:63–73.

13. Sparks CE, Sparks JD, Bolognino M, et al. Insulin effects on apolipoprotein B lipoprotein synthesis and secretion by primary cultures of rat hepatocytes. *Metabolism* 1986;35:1128–1136.

14. Pullinger CR, North JD, Teng B, et al. The apolipoprotein B gene is constitutively expressed in HepG2 cells: regulation of secretion by oleic acid, albumin, and insulin, and measurement of the mRNA half life. *J Lipid Res* 1989;30:1065–1077.

15. Sparks JD, Sparks CE, Miller LL. Insulin effects on apolipoprotein B production by normal, diabetic and treated-diabetic rat liver and cultured rat hepatocytes. *Biochem J* 1989;261:83–88.

16. Bartlett SM, Gibbons GF. Short- and longer-term regulation of very-low-density lipoprotein secretion by insulin, dexamethasone, and lipogenic substrates in cultured hepatocytes. *Biochem J* 1988;249:37–43.

17. Shumak SL, Zinman B, Zuniga-Guarjardo S, et al. Triglyceride-rich lipoprotein metabolism during acute hyperinsulinemia in hypertriglyceridemic humans. *Metabolism* 1988;37:461–466.

18. Alcindor L-G, Infante R, Soler-Argilaga C, Polonovski J. Effect of a single insulin administration on the hepatic release of triglyceride into the plasma. *Biochim Biophys Acta* 1973;306:347–352.

19. Topping DL, Trimble RP, Storer GB. Perfusate hematocrit value and insulin stimulation of lipogenesis and very low density lipoprotein secretion in perfused rat liver. *Biochem Int* 1981;3:101–106.

20. Storer GB, Trimble RP, Topping DL. Impaired sensitivity to insulin of rat livers perfused with blood of diminished haematocrit. *Biochem J* 1982;192:219–222.

Atherosclerosis Reviews, Volume 22,
edited by A. M. Gotto, Jr. and R. Paoletti.
Raven Press, Ltd., New York © 1991.

Sex Hormone Control of Triglyceride Metabolism

Robert H. Knopp

*Northwest Lipid Research Clinic, University of Washington,
Seattle, Washington, 98104*

The purpose of this brief review is to describe the effects of estrogens, progestins, and androgens on triglyceride (TG) metabolism. It will explore the effects of these individual sex steroid classes on TG metabolism via examples of sex-steroid-hormone–altered states and, finally, speculate on the significance of these alterations in TG metabolism to cardiovascular disease (CVD) risk.

A model for the effects of estrogen and estrogen plus progestin on lipoprotein metabolism is shown in Fig. 1. In general, the traffic in lipoprotein transport through the circulation is enhanced as a result of estrogen treatment. The clearance of circulating chylomicron remnants is enhanced in oral-contraceptive-steroid–treated individuals. Very-low-density lipoprotein (VLDL) production and VLDL remnant removal are enhanced with estrogen therapy. The same treatment increases low-density lipoprotein (LDL) receptor activity, which may explain the enhanced clearance of VLDL remnants. Estrogen decreases the activity of hepatic lipase (HTGL), which is associated with elevated high-density lipoprotein (HDL) cholesterol concentrations. Bile acid excretion is also enhanced by estrogen therapy.

When progestin is added to estrogen, effects opposite to estrogen are observed in terms of both plasma concentrations and mechanistic effects. Progestin counters the enhancing effect of estrogen on VLDL secretion, and plasma TG decline in this setting of combined hormone treatment. VLDL cholesterol concentrations increase relative to TG when certain androgenic progestins are coadministered with estrogen. In addition, there is evidence that progestins decrease the clearance of LDL, possibly by a down-regulation of the LDL receptor. HDL cholesterol levels decline as HTGL increases. This increase in hepatic lipase may also enhance the extent to which VLDL or remnant TG are removed by the liver.

Table 1 summarizes the available research on the effects of estrogens and progestins on VLDL metabolism. At least 11 studies of the question have shown that estrogen consistently enhances plasma TG, VLDL TG and apo-

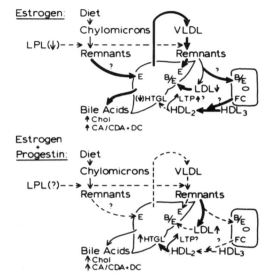

FIG. 1 Effects of estrogen and estrogen plus progestin on the lipoprotein cascade. An increased rate of traffic is indicated by the broad lines; a reduced rate of traffic is indicated by the dashed lines. In general, this model predicts an increase in traffic with estrogen treatment and the opposite effect with progestin.

protein secretion, and hepatic VLDL apoprotein mRNA levels (1–11). The effect of progesterone in combination with estrogen has been studied on three occasions. In 1975, Kim and Kalkhoff (3) found that estrogen plus progesterone slightly inhibited the entry of TG into the circulation in estrogen-treated rats using the Triton method of blocking lipoprotein lipase–mediated TG removal. On the other hand, in 1977 Chan and associates (5) found that progesterone did not oppose the estrogen enhancement of LDL entry into the circulation; but they only used a 2 to 1 M ratio of progesterone to estrogen, whereas Kim et al. used a $> 1,000$ to 1 M ratio. In 1981, Kenagy and associates confirmed that progesterone in a physiological molar ratio to estrogen ($> 1,000$ to 1) inhibited the estrogen-induced TG entry into the circulation (7). Other authors, including Chan et al. in 1978 (5), Capony and Williams in 1980 (9), Dashti et al. in 1983 (10), and Shaefer et al. in 1983 (11), all showed increases in VLDL apoprotein B (apoB) secretion with estrogen treatment.

Progestin inhibition of VLDL secretion in the absence of estrogen was reported by Wolfe and Grace in 1981 (12). In this study, norethindrone acetate inhibited TG fatty acid secretion in glucose-fed swine. Interestingly, however, when VLDL metabolism was evaluated in a hypertriglyceridemic subject given an anabolic androgen by Hazzard and associates (13), no reduction in VLDL secretion could be detected. Thus, the effect of androgenic steroids on VLDL secretion is unclear.

With respect to TG lipases, although administered estrogen has no effect on adipose tissue lipoprotein lipase (LPL) in humans, it leads to a consistent

TABLE 1. *Effects of estrogen on very-low-density lipoprotein (VLDL) triglyceride (TG) and apoprotein production*

Author	Yr	Journal	Medication (subjects)	Results
Kekki	1971	*Metabolism*	OCs	TG entry ↑
Glueck	1975	*Metabolism*	PM-ERT	TG entry ↑
Kim and Kalkhoff	1975	*J Clin Invest*	E_2 (rats)	TG entry ↑ ↑ [a]
			E_2 & P	TG entry ↑
Kudzma	1975	*J Lipid Res*	E_2 (chicks)	TG entry ↑
Chan et al.	1977	*Endocrinology*	E_2 (cockerels)	VLDL entry ↑ [b]
			E_2 & P (cockerels)	VLDL entry
			E_2 & P + nfx	VLDL entry
Weinstein	1978	*BBA*	E_2 (rats)	TG entry ↑ [a,c]
			F vs. M	TG entry ↑
Kenagy et al.	1981	*Endocrinology*	E_2 (rats)	TG entry ↑ ↑ [c]
			E_2 & P	TG entry ↑
Chan et al.	1978	*Circ Res*	E_2 (cockerels)[a]	Apo VLDL-II ↑
				Apo VLDL-II mRNA ↑
Capony and Williams	1980	*Biochemistry*	E_2 (roosters)	VLDL-apoB secretion ↑ [b]
Dashti et al.	1983	*J Lipid Res*	E_2 (turkeys)	Fatty acid synthesis ↑
				TG synthesis ↑
				VLDL apoB ↑
Schaefer et al.	1983	*J Clin Endocrinal Metab*	E_2 (young women)	VLDL-B SR ↑

[a] Triiton method.
[b] Liver slice secretion leucine labeled VLDL.
[c] Perfused liver secretion of triglyceride; L-CAT increased.

reduction in hepatic lipase (14). In addition, humans given anabolic steroids such as oxandrolone show an increase in hepatic lipase activity (15). The inverse association of hepatic lipase with HDL is well established (16). Different results have been observed in animal models (17), and an inverse association with adipose tissue LPL and endogenous plasma estrogen levels in obese women has been reported by Iverius and Brunzell (17).

The effects of sex steroids on remnant catabolism have been clearly delineated by the studies of estrogen treatment in type III hyperlipidemia where TG and cholesterol elevations are ameliorated with estrogen therapy (18) in association with enhanced remanent clearance (19). Surprisingly, however, in the d-norgestrel–treated rat, VLDL catabolism is also enhanced (20), possibly as a result of enhanced hepatic lipase activity. When postmenopausal women are given estrogen and d-norgestrel, an enhanced fractional catabolic rate of VLDL apoB is also observed (21), but in this human model, it is not clear if estrogenic or progestogenic mechanisms predominate. However, changes in VLDL lipid composition provide a clue to the significance of the hormone effects *in vivo*. For instance, we found that VLDL cholesterol concentrations for the amount of TG were increased in subjects taking an oral contraceptive steroid formulation containing a potent androgenic progestin (22). Conversely, Applebaum-Bowden and associates have found that estrogen therapy alone in cholesterol-fed postmenopausal women induces an increase in plasma VLDL TG concentrations with no VLDL cholesterol increase (23). Thus, as best as we can tell, estrogens have an anti-atherogenic effect on VLDL metabolism and composition whereas progestins and probably androgens have the opposite effect.

The relative effects of estrogens and natural progesterone or synthetic progestin on lipoproteins and vascular disease in oral contraceptive–using subjects, postmenopausal women, and pregnant lactating women have been compared in several reviews (24–27). One consistent feature of these hormone-induced effects is an increase in the TG content of LDL (26). It is unclear whether this effect is due to an increased activity of lipid transfer protein or if it reflects the enhanced rate of TG metabolism overall.

To analyze whether estrogen-induced effects on VLDL metabolism have significance for arteriosclerosis, one should consider the fact that VLDL cholesterol does not increase when estrogen treatment induces a VLDL TG rise (23). On the other hand, an androgenic oral contraceptive formulation increases VLDL cholesterol relative to TG (22). Finally, a reduction in cardiovascular disease risk is a consistent observation in over 25 studies of postmenopausal women treated with estrogen in case-control or cross-sectional studies, even where there is an increase in plasma TG (24,27). Although the beneficial effects of estrogen may be attributable to changes in LDL and HDL or a direct effect on the arterial wall, the increase in plasma TG concentrations certainly cannot be having a major detrimental effect.

In conclusion, estrogenic effects, including those on VLDL, seem to minimize arteriosclerosis risk; whereas potent androgenic progestins or androgens have the opposite effect. More studies are needed to clarify the effects of estrogens, progestins, and androgens on lipoprotein metabolism and CVD risk.

ACKNOWLEDGMENTS

This research was supported by the Clinical Nutrition Research Unit at the University of Washington, DK-35816.

REFERENCES

1. Kekki M, Nikkilä EA. Plasma triglyceride turnover during use of oral contraceptives. *Metabolism* 1971;20:878–889.
2. Glueck CJ, Fallat RW, Scheel D. Effects of estrogenic compounds on triglyceride kinetics. *Metabolism* 1975;24:537–545.
3. Kim H-J, Kalkhoff RK. Sex steroid influence on triglyceride metabolism. *J Clin Invest* 1975;56:888–896.
4. Kudzma DJ, St. Claire F, DeLallo L, Friedberg SJ. Mechanism of avian estrogen-induced

hypertriglyceridemia: evidence for overproduction of triglyceride. *J Lipid Res* 1975;16:123–133.

5. Chan L, Jackson RL, Means AR. Female steroid hormones and lipoprotein synthesis in the cockerel: effects of progesterone and nafoxidine on the estrogenic stimulation of very low density lipoproteins (VLDL) synthesis. *Endocrinology* 1977;100:1636–1643.

6. Weinstein I, Turner FC, Soler-Argilaga C, Heinberg M. Effects of ethinyl estradiol on serum lipoprotein lipids in male and female rats. *Biophys Acta* 1978;530:394–401.

7. Kenagy R, Weinstein I, Heimberg M. The effects of 17β-estradiol and progesterone on the metabolism of free fatty acid by perfused livers from normal female and ovariectomized rats. *Endocrinology* 1981;108:1614–1621.

8. Chan L, Jackson RL, Means AR. Regulation of lipoprotein synthesis: studies on the molecular mechanisms of lipoprotein synthesis and their regulation by estrogen in the cockerel. *Circ Res* 1978;43:209–217.

9. Capony F, Williams DL. Apolipoprotein B of avian very low density lipoprotein: characteristics of its regulation in nonstimulated and estrogen-stimulated rooster. *Biochemistry* 1980;19:2219–2226.

10. Dashti N, Kelley JL, Thayer RH, Ontko JA. Concurrent inductions of avian hepatic lipogenesis plasma lipids, and plasma apolipoprotein B by estrogen. *J Lipid Res* 1983;24:368–380.

11. Schaefer EJ, Foster DM, Zech LA, Lindgren FT, Brewer HB Jr., Levy RI. The effects of estrogen administration on plasma lipoprotein metabolism in premenopausal females. *J Clin Endocrinol Metab* 1983;57:262–267.

12. Wolfe BM, Grace DM. Norethindrone acetate inhibition of splanchnic triglyceride secretion in conscious glucose-fed swine. *J Lipid Res* 1979;20:175–182.

13. Hazzard WR, Kushwaha RS, Applebaum-Bowden D, et al. Chylomicron and very low-density lipoprotein apolipoprotein B metabolism: mechanism of the response to Stanozolol in a patient with severe hypertriglyceridemia. *Metabolism* 1984;33:873–881.

14. Applebaum DM, Goldberg AP, Pykalisto OJ, Brunzell JD, Hazzard WR. Effect of estrogen on post-heparin lipolytic activity: selective decline in hepatic triglyceride lipase. *J Clin Invest* 1977;59:601–608.

15. Enholm C, Huttenen JK, Kunnunen PJ, Nikkila EA. Effect of oxandrolone treatment on the activity of lipoprotein lipase, hepatic lipase and phoepholipase A, of human postheparin plasma. *N Engl J Med* 1975;292:1314–1317.

16. Tikkanen MJ, Nikkila EA. Regulation of hepatic lipase and serum lipoproteins by sex steroids. *Am Heart J* 1987;113:562–567.

17. Iverius PH, Brunzell JB. Relationship between lipoprotein lipase activity and plasma sex steroid levels in obese women. *J Clin Invest* 1988;82:1106–1112.

18. Hazzard WR. Primary type III hyperlipoproteinemia. In: Rifkind BM, Levy RI, eds. *Hyperlipidemia: diagnosis and therapy*. New York: Grune & Stratton, 1977;137–175.

19. Chait A, Albers JJ, Brunzell JD, Hazzard WR. Type III hyperlipoproteinemia ("remnant removal disease"). *Lancet* 1977;1:1176–1178.

20. Khokha R, Huff MW, Wolfe BM. Divergent effects of d-norgestrel on the metabolism of rat very low density and low density apolipoprotein B. *J Lipid Res* 1986;27:699–705.

21. Wolfe BM, Huff MW. Effects of combined estrogen and progestin administration on plasma lipoprotein metabolism in postmenopausal women. *J Clin Invest* 1989;83:40–45.

22. Knopp RH, Walden CE, Wahl PW, et al. Oral contraceptive and postmenopausal estrogen effects on lipoprotein triglyceride and cholesterol in an adult female population: relationships to estrogen and progestin potency. *J Clin Endocrinol Metab* 1981;53:1123–1132.

23. Applebaum-Bowden D, McLean P, Steinmetz A, et al. Lipoprotein, apolipoprotein, and lipolytic enzyme changes following estrogen administration in postmenopausal women. *J Lipid Res* 1989;30:1895–1906.

24. Knopp RH. Cardiovascular effects of endogenous and exogenous sex hormones over a woman's lifetime. *Am J Ob Gyn* 1988;158 (suppl 6):1630–1643.

25. Knopp RH, Warth MR, Childs CD, et al. Lipoprotein metabolism in pregnancy, fat transport to the fetus, and the effects of diabetes. *Biol Neonate (Paris)* 1986;50:297–317.

26. Knopp RH, Bergelin RO, Wahl PW, Walden CE. Effects of pregnancy, postpartum lactation and oral contraceptive use on the lipoprotein cholesterol/triglyceride ratio. *Metabolism* 1985;34:893–899.

27. Knopp RH. The effects of postmenopausal estrogen therapy on the incidence of arteriosclerotic vascular disease. *Obstet Gynecol* 1988;72:23S–30S.

Atherosclerosis Reviews, Volume 22,
edited by A. M. Gotto, Jr. and R. Paoletti.
Raven Press, Ltd., New York © 1991.

Diabetic Hypertriglyceridemia

Lipid and Lipoprotein Changes in Relation to Diabetes

Daniel Pometta and Richard W. James

*Division de Diabétologie, Hôpital Cantonal Universitaire,
Geneva CH-1211, Switzerland*

There are many factors that affect plasma lipids and the structure of lipoproteins in diabetes (Fig. 1), and thus contributing to hyperlipidemia. In particular, the quality of control of diabetes is critical; hyperlipidemia is often the clinical manifestation of poorly controlled diabetes. Genetic factors, such as the phenotype of apolipoprotein E (apoE), influence plasma triglyceride (TG) levels in diabetics; and triglyceridemia is also related to obesity, nephrotic syndrome, and kidney failure, all of which often complicate diabetes. Diet and alcohol consumption also help to determine plasma TG. Hypertriglyceridemia is the most frequent lipid disturbance in diabetes; it is not related to the severity of diabetes as measured by insulin dependence (1).

GENETIC INFLUENCE

The ApoE Phenotype

In nondiabetics, plasma lipids (2) and metabolic response to different diets (3) are influenced by the various phenotypes of apoE. Phenotype E 2/2 is the most frequent cause of dysbetalipoproteinemia in subjects with increased production of TG-rich lipoproteins (TGRL) (4). The substitution of a cysteine residue for arginine in position 158 of the apoE-3 molecule gives rise to the E2 isoform and also greatly reduces its binding to specific apoE receptors. Under normal conditions, even in the presence of the E2 phenotype, TGRL can be cleared from the system, but when very-low-density lipoprotein (VLDL) synthesis increases—a situation that occurs frequently in poorly controlled diabetes—this capacity is overwhelmed, so the concentration of TGRL increases in the blood (5). They are then diverted toward the mac-

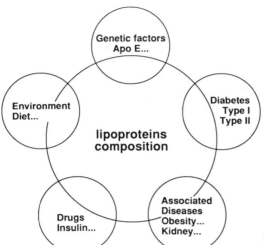

FIG. 1. Factors influencing lipoproteins composition in diabetics.

rophages; as they accumulate, they give rise to xanthomas and possibly to atherosclerosis.

The prevalence of the various apoE genotypes does not differ between the diabetic and nondiabetic populations (Table 1). Therefore, the increase of hypertriglyceridemia seen among diabetics cannot be attributed to greater apoE-2 mutation in their population (6).

However, in one group of poorly controlled diabetics examined by us (6), not only did the patients who displayed the homozygous E2 isoform have plasma cholesterol and TG above the 95th percentile limits (Table 2), they also had values significantly higher than diabetics with the more common E3/3 phenotype. When the patients carrying the apoE-2 allele (both homozygous and heterozygous) were considered together, their plasma triglycerides (2.72 mmol/L) were more elevated than those of diabetics carrying the E3 or E4 allele (1.88 mmol/L, $p < 0.05$).

ApoE is an example of a hereditary trait, inherited independently from diabetes, that affects the plasma lipid profile of diabetics. It may contribute to specific symptoms, such as the occurence of tuberous xanthomas (7) and the severity of coronary heart disease in diabetics carrying the E2 phenotype.

TABLE 1. *Frequency of E genotypes*

	Diabetics ($n = 195$)	Nondiabetics ($n = 173$)
$\Sigma 4$	0.097	0.107
$\Sigma 3$	0.813	0.821
$\Sigma 2$	0.090	0.072

TABLE 2. *Plasma lipids and apoE-2 and apoE-3 phenotypes*

Patients	E2/E2	E3/E2	E3/E3
Triglycerides (mmol/L)			
Diabetics	5.23 ± 2.21[a]	2.52 ± 2.17	1.87 ± 1.35
	(n = 4)	(n = 24)	(n = 132)
Nondiabetics	1.25 ± 0.3	1.41 ± 0.99	1.34 ± 0.69
	(n = 3)	(n = 12)	(n = 122)
Cholesterol (mmol/L)			
Diabetics	9.86 ± 4.35[a]	4.81 ± 1.44	5.0 ± 1.25
Nondiabetics	3.83 ± 0.98	4.72 ± 1.14	5.06 ± 1.33

[a] $p < 0.05$ in comparison to all other phenotypes.

LIPOPROTEIN COMPOSITION AND STRUCTURE

VLDL Composition in Poorly Controlled Type II Diabetics

Hypertriglyceridemia is a common feature of poorly controlled diabetes. It can often be corrected after 2 weeks of optimal diabetes control (8).

The composition of VLDL was studied in a group of hypertriglyceridemia type II diabetics who were normalized after 10 days of optimal treatment. Despite the lowering of patients' plasma cholesterol (6.3 ± 1.0 to 5.0 ± 0.6 mmol/L) and TG (4.7 ± 2.6 to 1.6 ± 0.4 mmol/L), the lipid composition of the VLDL expressed as a percentage of weight (Fig. 2) did not change. In contrast, the low apolipoprotein content (8) increased from 11.5% to 12.9% ($p < 0.01$) but still remained below the apolipoprotein content of the control group (13.9%).

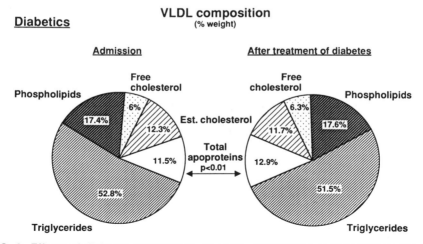

FIG. 2. Effects of diabetes equilibration on VLDL composition in hypertriglyceridemic patients.

The decrease in the VLDL apoprotein content, which is particularly marked in poorly controlled diabetics, is potentially dangerous because these particles are not as readily recognized by their specific receptors. This condition predisposes the patient to the development of premature coronary artery disease. The fact that reduction of the apoprotein content is associated with a decrease in the apoB content (8) is, in that respect, of major importance. It remains to be seen whether a more gradual equilibration of diabetes could fully normalize the VLDL apoprotein composition.

Lipoprotein Subfractions

The heterogeneity of VLDL and low-density lipoproteins (LDL) is well established. It has been attributed to discrete subpopulations of lipoprotein particles ($VLDL_1$–$VLDL_3$ and LDL_1–LDL_3) that differ in size, composition, and atherogenicity (9).

The effect of diabetes and diabetes equilibration on lipoprotein subfractions has been studied in both type I and type II diabetes. The lipoprotein subfractions were isolated by cumulative flotation ultracentrifugation in patients both at entry and after 10 days of hospitalization, when optimal control was established.

In type I diabetes (10), the plasma lipids (Table 3) appear within normal range. Nevertheless, a significant improvement in TG level was observed after 10 days of treatment. The lipoprotein subfraction distribution (Fig. 3) of poorly controlled type I diabetics shows a significant increase in $VLDL_2$ and $VLDL_3$; the latter are part of the intermediate-density lipoproteins (IDL) considered to be particularly atherogenic. As far as the LDL subclasses are concerned, LDL_3 are increased (10). LDL_3, in contrast to LDL_2, are lipoproteins that are poorly recognized by the LDL receptors and therefore potentially more atherogenic. Good control of diabetes reverses the subclasses' distribution to a pattern similar to the controls.

TABLE 3. *Male type I diabetic patients and controls: clinical characteristics*

Parameter	Diabetic patients ($n = 10$)		Controls ($n = 10$)
	Before	After	
Age (yr)	43.5 ± 10.6	—	42.7 ± 10.7
Plasma cholesterol (mm/L)	5.15 ± 0.97	4.70 ± 0.80	5.20 ± 0.65
Plasma TG (mm/L)	1.31 ± 0.51	0.96 ± 0.33[a]	1.11 ± 0.33
HDL-cholesterol (mm/L)	1.34 ± 0.25	1.23 ± 0.27[b]	1.19 ± 0.21[c]
ApoA-I (mg/dl)	151.4 ± 30.2	145.0 ± 30.6	149.6 ± 17.8
ApoB (mg/dl)	111.2 ± 15.5	92.8 ± 15.4	111.4 ± 33.7

[a] $p < 0.005$.
[b] $p < 0.02$.
[c] $p < 0.05$.

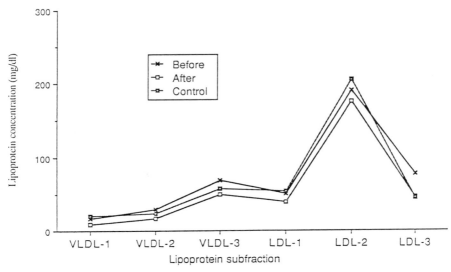

FIG. 3. Type I diabetes. Lipoprotein subfractions distribution before and after optimal equilibration.

Type II diabetics more frequently have abnormal plasma lipid patterns, but these too are readily corrected by improved diabetes control (Table 4). Our recent study of the lipoprotein subclass distribution (11) showed that poorly controlled diabetics had an increase of VLDL-1 to -3 subfractions and LDL$_3$ (Fig. 4), whereas LDL$_2$ were decreased. Significant improvement in the lipoprotein profile was obtained with diabetes equilibration over a period of 10 days, but complete normalization was not achieved. Indeed, the increase in VLDL$_3$ and LDL$_3$ was still evident. It is possible that a more

TABLE 4. *Male type II diabetic patients and controls: clinical characteristics*

Parameter	Diabetic patients ($n = 10$) Before	After	Controls ($n = 10$)
Age (yr)	54.3 ± 8.6	—	54.2 ± 7.9
Plasma cholesterol (mm/L)	$5.99 \pm 0.83^{a,b}$	5.13 ± 0.86	5.88 ± 0.75
Plasma TG (mm/L)	$3.09 \pm 0.87^{c,d}$	1.69 ± 0.50	1.05 ± 0.32
HDL-cholesterol (mm/L)	0.86 ± 0.10^{c}	0.84 ± 0.14^{c}	1.35 ± 0.34
ApoA-I (mg/dl)	146.7 ± 26.9^{e}	127.1 ± 24.4^{a}	168.9 ± 33.5
ApoB (mg/dl)	145.2 ± 19.1^{b}	119.1 ± 23.2	136.1 ± 38.7

[a] $p < 0.005$.
[b] $p < 0.005$.
[c] $p < 0.001$.
[d] $p < 0.001$ vs. posttreatment diabetic patients.
[e] $p < 0.05$.

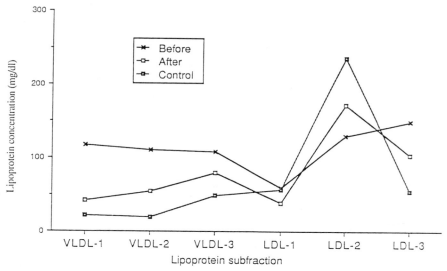

FIG. 4. Type II diabetes. Lipoprotein subfraction distribution before and after optimal equilibration.

prolonged period of treatment could fully normalize the lipoprotein subclass distribution.

CONCLUSION

Lipoprotein changes occurring in diabetes may have an adverse influence on the development of atherosclerosis. The various changes, particularly those in lipoprotein subclass distribution, are not always detectable by the measurement of plasma and HDL cholesterol or plasma TG. The potential for risk of coronary disease may be mitigated by improved diabetes control. At the same time, it should be understood that hereditary traits not related to diabetes, such as the apoE phenotype, may also affect plasma lipids and therefore promote the development of atherosclerosis.

ACKNOWLEDGMENTS

This study was supported by grants from the Swiss National Science Foundation (no. 3, 852-0.88) and the Swiss Diabetes Foundation.

REFERENCES

1. Pometta D. Insuffisance coronarienne, hyperlipémies et diabète. *Journ Annu Diebetol Hotel Dieu* 1976;20:249–257.

2. Sing CF, Davignon JM. Role of the apolipoprotein polymorphism in determining normal plasma lipid and lipoprotein variation. *Am J Hum Genet* 1985;37:268–285.
3. Tikkanen MJ, Huttunen JK, Ehnholm C, Pietinen P. Apolipoprotein E4 homozygosity predisposes to serum cholesterol elevation during high fat diet. *Arteriosclerosis* 1990;10:285–288.
4. Utermann G, Kindermann I, Kaffarnik H, Steinmetz A. Apolipoprotein E phenotypes and hyperlipidemia. *Hum Genet* 1984;65:232–236.
5. Utermann G, Hees M, Steinmetz A. Polymorphism of apo E and occurrence of dysbeta-lipoproteinemia in man. *Nature* 1977;269:604–607.
6. James RW, Voliotis C, Grab B, Pometta D. Phenotypes de l'approtéine E (apo E) et lipides sériques des diabétiques. *Schweiz Med Wochenschr* 1987;117:2021–2023.
7. Winocour PH, Tetlow L, Durrington PN, Ishola M, Hillier V, Anderson DC. Apolipoprotein E polymorphism and lipoproteins in insulin-treated diabetes mellitus. *Atherosclerosis* 1989;75:167–173.
8. Leowski J, James RW, Taton J, Pometta D. The influence of metabolic control on very low density lipoprotein composition in hypertriglyceridemic type II diabetics. A study using heparin-sepharose chromatography. *Metabolism* 1988;37:721–726.
9. Deckelbaum RJ, Granot E, Oschry Y, Rose L, Eisenberg S. Plasma triglyceride determines structure-composition in low and high density lipoproteins. *Arteriosclerosis* 1984;4:225–231.
10. James RW, Pometta D. Differences in lipoprotein subfraction composition and distribution between diabetic patients and controls. A study in male type 1 (insulin dependent) diabetes. *Diabetes* 1990;39:1158–1164.
11. James RW, Iometta D. The distribution profiles of very low density and low density lipoproteins in poorly controlled male, type 2 (non-insulin dependent) diabetic patients. *Diabetologia* 1991 (in press).

Atherosclerosis Reviews, Volume 22,
edited by A. M. Gotto, Jr. and R. Paoletti.
Raven Press, Ltd., New York © 1991.

Postprandial Dyslipidemia and Coronary Artery Disease

Josef R. Patsch

*Division of Clinical Atherosclerosis Research, Department of Medicine,
University of Innsbruck, A-6020 Innsbruck, Austria*

Several notable studies have used univariate analyses to correlate plasma triglycerides (TG) in postabsorptive plasma with the risk of coronary artery disease (CAD) (1–4). The relationship tends to break down when multivariate analyses are employed (5–8) because the TG are canceled out by the powerful risk factor high density lipoprotein (HDL) cholesterol (9,10). However, this elimination by statistical procedure does not necessarily disqualify TG-rich lipoproteins (TGRLP) as causative agents for CAD.

The levels of HDL cholesterol and TG are inversely associated because the metabolism of TGRLP determines HDL-cholesterol levels over a wide range (11). This relationship has been documented clearly for the postprandial state (11) where the entry of chylomicrons into the circulation challenges an individual's fat-clearing capacity.

The mechanisms underlying the negative association (10) between HDL cholesterol and CAD are obscure. Two principal scenarios have been proposed. In one of them, the "causalist" view, HDL are thought to trap excess cholesterol from cellular membranes by esterification. Transfer of the esterified cholesterol to TGRLP and subsequent removal by hepatic receptors completes the reverse cholesterol transport.

The alternative hypothesis, the "noncausalist" view, is based mainly on the negative association between the levels of HDL cholesterol and TG. This inverse relationship becomes even more pronounced when HDL levels, particularly those of HDL_2, are correlated with postprandial TG levels (11,12). In the noncausalist view, HDL do not interfere directly with cholesterol deposition and the arterial wall but rather reflect the ability of an individual to catabolize TGRLP in an efficient way.

Both the intimate relationship between the metabolism of TGRLP and HDL and the importance of chylomicron metabolism on HDL composition and levels (12,13) suggest that TG play an important role in the development of CAD in at least one of two ways: They could be atherogenic *per se*, and this atherogenicity could be signaled by low HDL levels, or they could be atherogenic due to their ability to decrease the levels of the powerful risk factor HDL cholesterol.

One potential reason for the failure of TG to constitute an independent risk factor for CAD is that TG metabolism cannot be well characterized by measuring fasting TG levels. Quantifying the degree of lipemia after a standardized oral fat load might constitute a more meaningful method of characterizing TG metabolism. Therefore, we set out to investigate whether TG metabolism as reflected in postprandial lipemia differs between CAD patients and controls. A clinical study was designed in which patients who underwent coronary arteriography and had fasting plasma TG of < 250 mg/dl were subjected to a fat tolerance test of 8 hr duration (11).

Patients with a coronary score of > 50 (i.e., severe CAD) were compared to control subjects with a coronary score of 0. A preliminary evaluation of 93 subjects from this ongoing study indicates that coronary patients differ from controls in their levels of fasting TG and HDL_2 cholesterol. The magnitude of postprandial lipemia is clearly and significantly larger in patients than in controls. When we considered all conventional lipid parameters for the fasting state, postprandial lipemia, quantified as the area under the postprandial TG curve, discriminated strongest between coronary cases and controls. In addition to the area under the 8-hr TG curve, single postprandial TG levels are also able to discriminate between cases and controls. Although early postprandial time points are not useful for discrimination, later time points beginning with 6 hr postprandially, discriminate between CAD cases and controls. Thus, the practicability of the fat load test of 8-hr duration and 2-hr blood drawings may be greatly enhanced in that only one or two postprandial blood specimens per fat load test may be needed. This simplification of the test would make it more useful for epidemiologic studies.

The preliminary data presented herein add to the accumulating evidence suggesting that TG should not be prematurely dismissed as an potential important risk factor for CAD (9). It is clear that there exists a relationship of different powers between TG, HLD cholesterol, and CAD risk, but when one considers the three together, the importance of individual correlates, as well as the mechanisms underlying these associations, is not very clear. However, there is a large body of evidence to suggest that the metabolism of TGRLP largely effects the plasma levels of HDL cholesterol, and that HDL cholesterol could be an integrative marker of TG transport in all states of absorption with the tendency to eliminate the fluctuating TG levels as a risk factor (14). The preliminary evidence presented in this article suggests that the metabolism of TGRLP when challenged by a standardized oral fat load may indeed be able to discriminate between CAD cases and controls, and may allow in the future to better evaluate the role of TGRLP in CAD.

ACKNOWLEDGMENT

This work was supported by grants HL-27341 from the National Institutes of Health and S-64/06 from the Austrian Fonds zur Förderung der Wissenschaftlichen Forschung.

REFERENCES

1. Carlson LA, Böttiger LE, Ahfeldt PE. Risk factors for myocardial infarction in the Stockholm prospective study: a 14-year follow-up focusing on the role of plasma triglycerides and cholesterol. *Acta Med Scand* 1979;206:351–360.
2. Brown DF. Blood lipids and lipoproteins in atherogenesis. *Am J Med* 1969;46:691–704.
3. Brunner D, Altmann S, Loebl K. et al. Serum cholesterol and triglycerides in patients suffering from ischemic heart disease and in healthy subjects. *Atherosclerosis* 1977;28:197–204.
4. Carlson LA, Böttiger LE. Ischemic heart disease in relationship to testing values of plasma triglycerides and cholesterol. *Lancet* 1972;1:865–868.
5. Hulley SB, Rosenmann RH, Bavol RD, et al. Epidemiology as a guide to clinical decisions: the association between triglyceride and coronary heart disease. *N Engl J Med* 1980;302:1383–1389.
6. Heyden S, Heiss G, Hames CG, at el. Fasting triglycerides as predictors of total and CHD mortality in Evans County, Georgia. *J Chronic Dis* 1980;33:275–282.
7. Castelli WP, Doyle JT, Gordon T, et al. HDL cholesterol and other lipids in coronary heart disease: the cooperative lipoprotein phenotyping study. *Circulation* 1977;55:767–772.
8. Lewis B, Chait A, Oakley CM, et al. Serum lipoprotein abnormalities in patients with ischemic heart disease: comparisons with a control population. *Brit Med J* 1974;3:489–493.
9. Austin ME. Plasma triglyceride as a risk factor for coronary heart disease. The epidemiologic evidence and beyond. *Am J Epidemiol* 1989;129:249–259.
10. Tyroler HA. Epidemiology of plasma high-density lipoprotein cholesterol levels. *Circulation* 1980;62 (suppl IV):IV1–IV3.
11. Patsch Jr, Karlin JB, Scott LW, Gotto AM Jr. Inverse relationship between blood levels of high density lipoprotein subfraction 2 and magnitude of postprandial lipemia. *Proc Natl Acad Sci (USA)* 1983;80:1449–1453.
12. Patsch JR, Prasad S, Gotto AM Jr, Patsch W. High density lipoprotein 2: relationship of the plasma levels of this lipoprotein species to its composition, to the magnitude of postprandial lipemia and to the activities of lipoprotein lipase and hepatic lipase. *J Clin Invest* 1987;80:341–347.
13. Patsch JR, Prasad S, Gotto AM Jr, Bengtsson-Olivecrona G. Postprandial lipemia: a key for the conversion of HDL-2 into HDL-3 by hepatic lipase. *J Clin Invest* 1984;74:2017–2023.
14. Miesenböck G, Patsch JR. Relationship of triglyceride and high density lipoprotein metabolism. *Atherosclerosis Rev* 1990;18:119–128.

Atherosclerosis Reviews, Volume 22,
edited by A. M. Gotto, Jr. and R. Paoletti.
Raven Press, Ltd., New York © 1991.

Triglycerides and Atherosclerosis

Results from the Prospective Cardiovascular Münster Study

*†Gerd Assmann and †Helmut Schulte

*Institut für Klinische Chemie und Laboratoriumsmedizin, Zentrallaboratorium
der Universität Münster, †Institut für Arteriosklerose forschung an der
Universität Münster, D-4400 Münster, F.R.G.

Although the causal connection between hypercholesterolemia and athero-sclerosis is generally accepted and our understanding of the underlying mechanisms has progressed, the pathophysiological significance of hyper-triglyceridemia as a risk factor for atherosclerosis remains unclear. One reason for this is that hypertriglyceridemia can reflect an increase in con-centration of any of several lipoproteins that play different roles in ather-ogenesis—i.e., chylomicrons, the various subclasses of very-low-density lipoprotein (VLDL), and intermediate-density lipoprotein (IDL). Another is that increases in the concentration of triglyceride-rich lipoprotein (TGRLP) can result from disturbances of lipoprotein metabolism that may well differ in their bearing on atherogenesis. There is reason to suspect that certain subgroups of lipoproteins with a high triglyceride (TG) content play a casual role in atherosclerosis, but studies of the status of TGRLP as independent predictors of coronary heart disease (CHD) risk have yielded contradictory results.

The still-controversial status of TG as a risk factor in CHD is illustrated by the recently published strategy paper of the European Atherosclerosis Society (EAS) on the primary prevention of coronary heart disease (1). Al-though this group recognizes that many causes of hypertriglyceridemia re-quire treatment in their own right (e.g., obesity, alcohol abuse, and untreated diabetes mellitus), the EAS consensus view is that the data now available are not adequate to establish firm guidelines for TG determination in the assessment of CHD risk or for the treatment of elevated plasma TG to reduce this risk. Moreover, the strategy paper contends that the predictive value of TG concentration is diminished by its considerable variation over the course of the day. The EAS recommends that TG be measured in the fasting state. An American group has advised that levels > 5.6 mmol/L require active therapy and has recommended treatment for levels > 11 mmol/L to lessen the risk of pancreatis (2).

In consideration of these issues, and to demonstrate the relationship between TG and risk of CHD, some results of the Prospective Cardiovascular Münster (PROCAM) study are presented here.

DESCRIPTION OF THE PROCAM STUDY

In the PROCAM study, employees of 52 different organizations were first examined for cardiovascular risk factors, then kept under observation to record all deaths as well as new myocardial infarctions (MI) and strokes. The examination at entry into the program consisted of an anamnesis using standardized questionnaires, measurement of blood pressure and anthropometric data, a resting electrocardiographic tracing (ECG), and collection of a blood sample after a 12-hr fast for the determination of more than 20 laboratory parameters. The methods used for the examinations (3) and the laboratory tests (4) are described in detail elsewhere.

The examination was carried out in a converted bus on the employer's site during paid working hours. Any employee could participate in the study. Participation was voluntary; between 40% and 80% of employees took part (average, 60%). The program was free of charge to both the volunteers and their employers (apart from loss of work). About 20 people were examined per day. All findings were reported to the participant's general practitioner. He or she was told whether the results of the examination were normal, or whether a check-up by the general practitioner was necessary. We ourselves neither carried out nor arranged for any intervention; this was left to the individual's general practitioner.

Questionnaires were then sent to the participants every 2 years to record any MI or strokes that occurred in the meantime and also to find out about any deaths. At the initial examination, participants were told to complete a questionnaire every 2 years. The response rate was 96% after two reminders by mail and phone each if necessary. For all deaths and also any other incidents reported in the questionnaire, we requested hospital records and records from the attending physician in order to verify the diagnosis or the cause of death. Surviving patients were first asked for their permission. The initial examination will be repeated after 6 to 7 years.

A total of 19,698 men and women were enrolled between 1979 and 1985. The ages ranged from 16 to 65 years. The average age of the 13,737 men was 41.4 years ± 11.2 years. The 5,961 women had a distinctly lower age of 36.6 ± 12.5 years.

TABLE 1. *PROCAM study: mean values of triglycerides according to age[a]*

Age (yr)	Men	Women
16–25	97 (5,6)	85 (2,2)
26–35	133 (14,8)	90 (3,6)
36–45	165 (21,2)	95 (4,2)
46–55	164 (21,7)	106 (5,6)
56–65	150 (19,2)	122 (7,9)

[a] The figures in parentheses represent percentages of individuals with triglycerides $\geq$ 200 mg/dl.

PREVALENCE DATA FROM PROCAM

Mean values of TG are higher in men than in women. Triglycerides increased linearly with age in women. In men, they increased up to the age of 35 years, remained constant for ages 35 through 55 years, and decreased thereafter (Table 1). According to these findings, hypertriglyceridemia (defined as TG $\geq$ 200 mg/dl) was much more common among men (18.6%) than women (4.2%). Prevalence increased with age in women, but remained nearly constant at about 20% in men aged 35 years or more.

In a subgroup of 864 men and 373 women, the following coagulation parameters were also determined: fibrinogen, factor VII, antithrombin III, protein C, and plasminogen activator inhibitor type 1 activity (PAI-1). Baseline population characteristics are given in Table 2.

To analyze the relationship between TG and significant parameters in CHD, we performed a multiple regression analysis on log-transformed values of TG, as TG are log-normally distributed. Both men and women showed a strong negative correlation between TG and HDL cholesterol (Table 3). A positive relationship was observed in both sexes with cholesterol, blood glucose, factor VIIc, and PAI-1. In men only, TG are positively correlated with apoA-I, body mass index, cigarette smoking, and alcohol consumption (Table 3). Postmenopausal woman showed higher triglyceride values than premenopausal women. No independent relationships were observed to age, blood pressure, apolipoprotein (a) [Lp (a)], apoA-II, apoB, AT-III, protein C, fibrinogen, or oral contraceptives.

INCIDENCE OF CHD ACCORDING TO TG

Over an observation period of 4 years, 73 episodes of MI and fatal coronary events occurred among 2754 male participants aged 40 to 65 years who had no prior history of MI or stroke. The 2,681 subjects not affected by MI or

TABLE 2. PROCAM study: population characteristics (mean values ± SD) of subgroup with coagulation parameters

	Men (n = 864)	Women (n = 373)
Age (yr)	43.2 ± 11.3	38.6 ± 11.8
Systolic blood pressure (mm Hg)	127.0 ± 15.1	122.6 ± 14.5
Body mass index (kg/m²)	25.6 ± 3.2	23.8 ± 4.0
Cholesterol (mg/dl)	212.2 ± 41.3	207.3 ± 36.8
HDL cholesterol (mg/dl)	46.1 ± 11.6	59.8 ± 15.5
LDL cholesterol (mg/dl)	139.6 ± 37.3	127.4 ± 35.5
Triglycerides (mg/dl)	135.9 ± 94.5	100.6 ± 55.5
ApoA-I (mg/dl)	140.2 ± 20.7	159.9 ± 26.4
ApoA-II (mg/dl)	43.1 ± 7.2	43.6 ± 8.3
ApoB (mg/dl)	87.4 ± 21.4	77.9 ± 19.6
Apolipoprotein(a) (mg/dl)	16.4 ± 24.6	16.4 ± 27.1
Blood glucose (mg/dl)	99.2 ± 16.3	94.0 ± 15.3
Alcohol consumption (g/day)	10.1 ± 15.4	1.9 ± 0.3
Fibrinogen (mg/dl)	266.3 ± 59.1	270.7 ± 57.0
Factor VII (%)	104.0 ± 23.7	111.9 ± 28.8
AT-III (%)	99.0 ± 10.4	99.2 ± 10.9
PAI-1 (U/ml)	3.7 ± 2.9	2.7 ± 2.4
Protein C (%)	100.7 ± 16.9	101.4 ± 18.7
Current cigarette smokers (%)	28.5	33.5
Oral contraceptives users (%)		24.9
Postmenopausal women (%)		27.1

fatal CHD (MI−) had a mean TG level of 160.4 mg/dl (median, 130.7 mg/dl); whereas in victims of MI or fatal CHD (MI+), the mean concentration was 178.6 mg/dl (median, 155.8 mg/dl). In the MI–group, 21.0% of participants had TG > 200 mg/dl; in the MI+ group, 31.5% of subjects exceeded this limit (5). The numbers of observed CHD events per tertile of

TABLE 3. PROCAM study: multiple regression of triglycerides (logarithm)

	Standardized regression coefficients	
	Male (n = 864)	Female (n = 373)
HDL cholesterol	−0.55***	−0.45***
Cholesterol	0.37***	0.27***
PAI-1	0.23***	0.20***
ApoA-I	0.16***	0.04
Body mass index	0.10***	0.08
Factor VIIc	0.09**	0.23***
Alcohol consumption	0.05*	0.05
Blood glucose	0.05*	0.12**
Smoking	0.05*	0.01
Menopause	—	0.11*

No significant relationship to age, blood pressure, Lp(a), apoA-II, apoB, oral contraceptives, AT-III, protein C, fibrinogen.
*p <0.05, **p <0.01, ***p <0.0001.

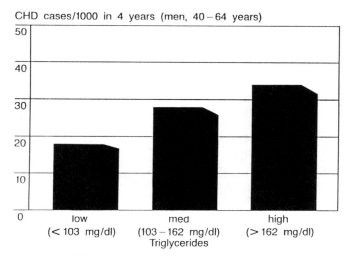

CHD cases/1000 in 4 years (men, 40 – 64 years)

low
(< 103 mg/dl)

med
(103 – 162 mg/dl)
Triglycerides

high
(> 162 mg/dl)

FIG. 1. PROCAM study: CHD incidence according to triglycerides.

the TG distribution were 18, 28, and 34 per 1,000 subjects within 4 years, respectively (Fig. 1). However, in a multivariate analysis by means of a multiple logistic function taking into account the parameters of age, HDL cholesterol, cholesterol, systolic blood pressure, diabetes mellitus, MI in the family, and angina pectoris, the association between TG and CHD disappeared (6).

A projected slope analysis of the Framingham Study (7) has revealed TG as an independent CHD risk factor in men over 50 years of age, particularly those with low HDL cholesterol or with high total cholesterol/HDL cholesterol ratios (8).

A breakdown of CHD incidence rates in the PROCAM study by tertiles of HDL cholesterol and TG (Fig. 2) showed a slight increase of CHD rates with increasing TG within each HDL cholesterol tertile.

The subgroup of PROCAM participants with high total cholesterol/HDL cholesterol ratios (> 5.0) showed an increased risk of CHD (42/1,000 subjects in 4 years) compared to men with low ratios (9/1,000 subjects in 4 years) (Fig. 3). In particular those men with high total cholesterol/HDL cholesterol ratios based upon low HDL cholesterol levels (< 35 mg/dl) had a higher risk for CHD (incidence rate, 91/1,000 subjects in 4 years) than men with high ratios but high HDL cholesterol levels (incidence rate, 15/1,000 subjects in 4 years). The latter subgroup showed no relationship between CHD risk and TG (Fig. 3). In contrast, in men with high total cholesterol/HDL cholesterol ratios and low HDL cholesterol levels, hypertriglyceridemia is an additional risk factor for CHD.

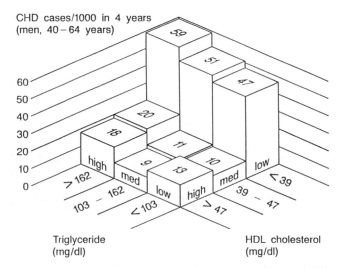

FIG. 2. PROCAM study: CHD incidence according to triglycerides and HDL cholesterol.

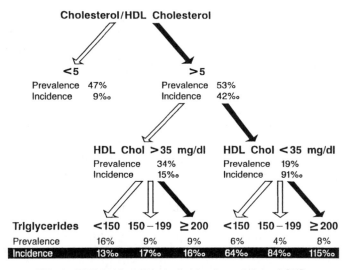

FIG. 3. PROCAM study: dyslipidemia and risk of CHD.

SUMMARY

In the PROCAM study, hypertriglyceridemia was far more common among men (18.6%) than women (4.2%). Whereas its prevalence increased with age in women, it remained nearly constant (at ~20%) in men aged ≥ 35.

A multiple regression analysis yielded a strong negative correlation between TG and HDL cholesterol. In both sexes, a positive relationship was observed with cholesterol, blood glucose, factor VIIc, and PAI-1. In men only, TG are positivly correlated with apoA-I, body mass index, cigarette smoking, and alcohol consumption. Postmenopausal women showed higher TG levels than premenopausal women. No independent relationships were observed to age, blood pressure, Lp(a), apoA-II, apoB, AT-III, protein C, fibrinogen, and oral contraceptives.

The PROCAM study did not identify TG as an independent risk factor, but the data suggest that hypertriglyceridemia is an additional risk factor for CHD when excessive TG coincide with a high ratio of plasma cholesterol to HDL cholesterol and with low HDL cholesterol values.

ACKNOWLEDGMENTS

This work has been supported by the Bundesministerium für Forschung und Technologie, Ministerium für Wissenschaft und Forschung NRW, Deutsche Forschungsgemeinschaft, and Landesversicherungsanstalt (LVA) Westfalen.

REFERENCES

1. Study Group, European Atherosclerosis Society. Strategies for the prevention of coronary heart disease: a policy statement of the European Atherosclerosis Society. *Eur Heart J* 1987;8:77–88.
2. Consensus conference. Treatment of hypertriglyceridaemia. *JAMA* 1984;251:1196–1200.
3. Assmann G, Schulte H. *Procam-Studie*. Hedingen Zürich: Panscientia Verlag, 1986.
4. Assmann G, Oberwittler W, Schulte H, et al. Prädiktion and Frükerkennung der koronaren Herzkrankheit. *Internist* 1980;21:446–459.
5. Schulte H, Assmann G. Ergebnisse der "Prospective Cardiovascular Muenster" (PROCAM)-Studie. *Soz Praventivmed* 1988;33:32–36.
6. Assmann G, Schulte H. The Prospective Cardiovascular Muenster (PROCAM) study: prevalence of hyperlipidemia in persons with hypertension and/or diabetes mellitus and the relationship to coronary heart disease. *Am Heart J* 1988;116:1713–1724.
7. Abbot RD, Carrol R. Interpreting multiple logistic regression coefficients in prospective observational studies. *Am J Epidemiol* 1984;119:830–836.
8. Castelli WP. The triglyceride issue: a view from Framingham. *Am Heart J* 1986;112:432–437.

Atherosclerosis Reviews, Volume 22,
edited by A. M. Gotto, Jr. and R. Paoletti.
Raven Press, Ltd., New York © 1991.

The Impact of Triglycerides on Coronary Heart Disease

The Framingham Study

Peter W. F. Wilson, Keaven M. Anderson, and William P. Castelli

Framingham Heart Study, Framingham, Massachusetts 01701

The association of triglyceride (TG) levels with coronary heart disease (CHD) continues to be debated (1–3). In general, TGs are associated with coronary disease in many long-term studies. Triglyceride-lowering with pharmacologic agents in secondary prevention trials has been associated with lower CHD rates (4,5), but the high inverse correlation of TG levels with high-density lipoprotein (HDL)-cholesterol clouds the picture.

MATERIALS AND METHODS

Data for this report are based on information from lipid measurements made on the Framingham cohort in 1952–54, 1966–68, and 1972–74. Determinations were made using the Svedberg fraction (S_f) technique in a collaborative effort with the Donner Laboratories at biennial exam two in 1952–54 (6), nonfasting TG levels at biennial exam eight in 1966–68, and fasting TG at biennial exam 11 in 1972–74. Patients were nonfasting for the 1952–54 and 1966–68 determinations and fasting at the 1972–74 exam. At the 1966–68 and the 1972–74 exams, the Kessler technique was used for measurement of TG (7). Lipoprotein cholesterol fractions were first determined on the heart study cohort in 1972–74, after a modification of the Lipid Research Clinic's protocol, using heparin-manganese precipitation (8). Because all lipid measurements were made at regular clinic visits, information on age, height, weight, cigarette smoking during the past year, blood pressure determinations, blood cholesterol level, glucose intolerance, and electrocardiographic left ventricular hypertrophy were also available (9).

After participants with prevalent CHD [angina pectoris, myocardial infarction (MI), or coronary insufficiency] at the baseline examinations were excluded from the analyses, patients were followed for the incidence of cardiovascular events. Proportional hazards regression was used in some analyses with the independent variable of TG accompanied only by age. In multivariate analyses, the variables included age, TG levels, systolic blood pressure, total blood cholesterol, number of cigarettes smoked per day in the year prior to examination, glucose intolerance, body mass index, and left ventricular hypertrophy on the electrocardiogram.

RESULTS

Table 1 demonstrates the relationship between S_f 20 to 400 concentrations in the plasma with later CHD. This TG-rich plasma fraction was strongly associated with CHD in age-adjusted analyses. However, the correlation was weakened moderately in women and considerably in men when a full multivariate model was run and adjustment was made for blood cholesterol and the other cardiovascular risk factors.

The association between TG and CHD for individuals free of CHD at biennial exam seven (1964–66) is shown in Table 2, according to TG levels. After age adjustment, these nonfasting TG levels were associated with increased CHD in women, but the effect in men was borderline ($p = 0.08$). Multivariate adjustment weakened the associations, particularly in men. Nonfasting TG were repeated 2 years later, at the 1966–68 exam. The associations with CHD were much stronger, as seen in Table 3.

Table 4 shows the association between CHD and fasting TG measured at the 11th biennial exam in 1972–74. After age adjustment, the TG levels are associated with CHD in women but not in men. Cholesterol and HDL cholesterol were also measured at this exam. The relationships between the various lipid measures, either singly or in combination with CHD, are shown in Tables 5 and 6 for men and women, respectively. The hazard ratio is computed by first multiplying the β estimated from the proportional hazards model by the number of units listed. Subsequently, this value is exponentiated to get an estimate of the "hazard ratio" associated with the stated measurement difference. An estimate of the hazard ratio is analogous to the odds, or risk, ratio. This calculation procedure is repeated using endpoints of a confidence interval for β to obtain a confidence interval for the hazard ratio (10).

DISCUSSION

The following issues should be considered in any discussion of the relationship between TG and CHD: age and gender of participants, fasting versus nonfasting samples, and availability of other covariates. At the time of the earliest TG measurements for the heart study, the participants were middle-aged and nonfasting. Among both sexes, the TG levels were predictive of

TABLE 1. Thirty-two-year age-adjusted incidence of CHD according to nonfasting S_f 20–400 fractions, Framingham cohort 35–84, follow-up 1954–1986

Men		Women	
S_f 20–400 (mg/dl)	Rate (per 1,000/10 yr)	S_f 20–400 (mg/dl)	Rate (per 1,000/10 yr)
<100	71	<50	29
100–149	99	50–89	31
150–199	98	90–129	41
200–249	149	130–169	62
>249	175	>169	52
At risk	1,754		2,203
Cases	699		529
Age-adjusted test for trend	$p = 0.0001$		$p = 0.0001$
Multivariate-adjusted test for trend	$p = 0.6708$		$p = 0.0055$

TABLE 2. Twenty-two-year age-adjusted incidence of CHD according to nonfasting triglycerides, Framingham cohort 35–84, follow-up 1964–1986

Men		Women	
Triglycerides (mg/dl)	Rate (per 1,000/10 yr)	Triglycerides (mg/dl)	Rate (per 1,000/10 yr)
<100	113	<80	74
100–139	169	80–109	85
140–179	214	110–139	88
180–219	237	140–169	130
>220	195	>170	147
At risk	1,400		1,940
Cases	452		387
Age-adjusted test for trend	$p = 0.0859$		$p = 0.0001$
Multivariate-adjusted test for trend	$p = 0.9270$		$p = 0.0541$

TABLE 3. Twenty-year age-adjusted incidence of CHD according to nonfasting triglycerides, Framingham cohort 35–84, follow-up 1966–1986

Men		Women	
Triglycerides (mg/dl)	Rate (per 1,000/10 yr)	Triglycerides (mg/dl)	Rate (per 1,000/10 yr)
<50	154	<50	76
50–64	159	50–64	78
65–79	238	65–79	110
80–94	228	80–94	116
>94	217	>94	152
At risk	867		1,215
Cases	288		234
Age-adjusted test for trend	$p = 0.0019$		$p = 0.0024$
Multivariate-adjusted test for trend	$p = 0.0389$		$p = 0.1187$

TABLE 4. *Fourteen-year age-adjusted incidence of CHD according to fasting triglycerides, Framingham cohort 45–84, follow-up 1972–1986*

Men		Women	
Triglycerides (mg/dl)	Rate (per 1,000/10 yr)	Triglycerides (mg/dl)	Rate (per 1,000/10 yr)
<80	190	<70	74
80–109	169	70–99	107
110–139	257	100–129	115
140–159	273	130–159	160
>159	345	>159	170
At risk	935		1,317
Cases	232		203
Age-adjusted test for trend	$p = 0.4147$		$p = 0.0050$

TABLE 5. *Hazard ratios for CHD according to fasting lipids, Framingham cohort 45–84, follow-up 1972–1986, men*

Model	Cholesterol (10 mg/dl)		Triglycerides (40 mg/dl)		HDL-C (5 mg/dl)	
	Hazard ratio	(Confidence interval)	Hazard ratio	(Confidence interval)	Hazard ratio	(Confidence interval)
1	1.04	$(1.01–1.07)^a$				
2			1.00	(0.99–1.06)		
3					0.91	$(0.86–0.96)^b$
4	1.04	$(1.01–1.07)^a$	1.00	(0.99–1.01)		
5	1.04	$(1.01–1.07)^b$			0.90	$(0.85–0.95)^c$
6			1.00	(0.99–1.00)	0.91	$(0.86–0.96)^c$
7	1.05	$(1.02–1.08)^b$	1.00	(0.95–1.05)	0.89	$(0.84–0.95)^c$

Odds entries represent estimated change in risk associated with specified number of mg/dl for lipid measure. The 5% to 95% confidence intervals of the estimates are given in parentheses. All models include age adjustment.
[a] $0.01 < p < 0.05.$
[b] $0.001 < p < 0.01.$
[c] $p < 0.001.$

TABLE 6. *Hazard ratios for CHD according to fasting lipids, Framingham cohort 45–84, follow-up 1972–1986, women*

Model	Cholesterol (10 mg/dl)		Triglycerides (40 mg/dl)		HDL-C (5 mg/dl)	
	Hazard ratio	(Confidence interval)	Hazard ratio	(Confidence interval)	Hazard ratio	(Confidence interval)
1	1.05	$(1.02–1.09)^a$				
2			1.01	$(1.00–1.02)^a$		
3					0.90	$(0.85–0.94)^b$
4	1.04	$(1.01–1.08)^a$	1.01	$(1.00–1.01)^b$		
5	1.05	$(1.02–1.09)^b$			0.89	$(0.85–0.95)^b$
6			0.99	(0.99–1.00)	0.90	$(0.85–0.95)^b$
7	1.06	$(1.03–1.10)^b$	1.00	(0.99–1.01)	0.89	$(0.84–0.94)^b$

Odds entries represent estimated change in risk associated with specified number of mg/dl for lipid measure. The 5% to 95% confidence intervals of the estimates are given in parentheses. All models include age adjustment.
[a] $0.001 < p < 0.01.$
[b] $p < 0.001.$

CHD under these circumstances. Later TG determinations, such as those made at exam 11 in 1972–74, when all participants were > 50 years old, showed weaker relationships between TG levels and CHD, particularly after cholesterol of HDL cholesterol was taken into account in the statistical models.

Observational studies focus on the experience of the majority, and in most instances lipid levels do not differ greatly from the mean. However, the situation would be quite different for individuals with high TG levels. In such cases, pharmacological intervention might be initiated to prevent either an occurrence (11) or a recurrence of CHD (4,5).

Finally, covariates of higher TG should be considered as a part of the puzzle surrounding coronary disease. Individuals with high TG levels are most likely to have glucose intolerance and higher insulin levels (12,13). Either of these metabolic derangements could contribute to greater CHD risk independently of the TG level alone.

REFERENCES

1. Hulley SB, Rosenman RH, Bawol RD, Brand RJ. Epidemiology as a guide to clinical decisions. *N Engl J Med* 1980;302:1383–1389.
2. Castelli WP. Cholesterol and lipids in the risk of coronary artery disease—the Framingham Heart Study. *Can J Cardiol* 1988;4:5–10.
3. Freedman DS, Gruchow HW, Anderson AJ, Rimm AA, Barboriak JJ. Relation of triglyceride levels to coronary artery disease: the Milwaukee Cardiovascular Data Registry. *Am J Epidemiol* 1988;127:1118–1130.
4. Carlson LA, Rosenhamer G. Reduction of mortality in the Stockholm Ischaemic Heart Disease Secondary Prevention Study by combined treatment with clofibrate and nicotinic acid. *Acta Med Scand* 1988;223:405–418.
5. Canner PL, Berge KG, Wenger NK, et al. Fifteen year mortality in Coronary Drug Project patients: long-term benefit with niacin. *J Am Coll Cardiol* 1986;8:1245–1255.
6. Gofman JW, Hanig M, Jones HB, et al. Evaluation of serum lipoprotein and cholesterol measurements as predictors of clinical complications of atherosclerosis: report of a cooperative study of lipoproteins and atherosclerosis. *Circulation* 1956;14:691–741.
7. Kessler G, Lederer H. Fluorometric measurements of triglycerides. In: Skeggs LT, ed. *Technicon symposia automation in analytical chemistry.* New York: 1965:341–344.
8. Lipid Research Clinics Program. *Manual of laboratory operations; vol 1: Lipid and lipoprotein analysis.* DHEW publ. no (NIH) 75–628. Bethesda, Md.: National Institutes of Health, 1974.
9. Cupples LA, Ramaswamy R, Christiansen J, Belanger A, D'Agostino RB. The relationship between sporadically measured variables and the risk of cardiovascular disease and death: Framingham Heart Study, 30–34 year follow-up. *NTIS monograph,* 1988:1–20.
10. Cox DR. Regression models and life tables. *J R Stat Soc* 1972;34:187–220.
11. Frick MH, Elo O, Haapa K, et al. Helsinki Heart Study: primary prevention trial with gemfibrozil in middle-aged men with dyslipidemia. *N Engl J Med* 1987;317:1237–1245.
12. Wilson PWF, Kannel WB, Anderson KM. Lipids, glucose intolerance and vascular disease: the Framingham Study. Basel: Karger, 1985:1–11. (Karger monographs on atherosclerosis: vol 13. Dyslipidemias and diabetes.)
13. Zavaroni I, Bonora E, Pagliara M, et al. Risk factors for coronary artery disease in healthy persons with hyperinsulinemia and normal glucose tolerance. *N Engl J Med* 1989;320:702–706.

Atherosclerosis Reviews, Volume 22,
edited by A. M. Gotto, Jr. and R. Paoletti.
Raven Press, Ltd., New York © 1991.

Triglycerides and Coronary Heart Disease

Epidemiologic, Statistical, and Genetic Issues

Melissa A. Austin

*Department of Epidemiology, School of Public Health and Community Medicine,
University of Washington, Seattle, Washington, 98195*

The controversy over whether elevated plasma triglyceride (TG) levels are a risk factor for coronary heart disease (CHD) is ongoing. In order to gain some insights into the problem, we addressed three specific topics. First, we used observational epidemiologic studies to consider whether elevated plasma TG is associated with an increased risk of coronary heart disease. Second, because the results of the statistical analyses based on the epidemiologic data are often contradictory, we deemed it important to ask whether multivariate statistical analyses accurately estimates the association between TG and disease. Finally, in interpreting the epidemiologic results, we also asked whether there might be subgroups of genetically susceptible individuals. That is, are there individual patients in whom a genetically influenced mechanism is operating such that hypertriglyceridemia does increase risk of CHD?

OBSERVATIONAL EPIDEMIOLOGIC STUDIES

Most studies of the relationship between plasma TG levels and CHD have focused on men. The first study to report an association between increased TG levels and myocardial infarction (MI) was reported by Albrink and Man in 1959 (1). Since that time, at least 16 additional studies using either a retrospective or cross-sectional design and comparing cases with controls have been reported. With one exception—an international ecological study (2)—all have reported a significant univariate association. Several of these studies also considered whether the TG association with disease was independent of other lipid measures, using either stratification or multivariate statistical analysis techniques. All six of the studies that evaluated TG levels controlling for either total cholesterol or low-density lipoprotein (LDL) cholesterol levels found that the association of TG with disease persisted. Only four case-control studies in men adjusted for high-density lipoprotein (HDL) cholesterol. In three of these studies, the TG association remained; the exception was the Cooperative Lipoprotein Phenotyping Study (3).

An additional 16 studies used coronary angiography to assess the severity of coronary heart disease in relation to TG levels in men. In general, these studies have also demonstrated a univariate association, the most recent being a report from the Milwaukee Cardiovascular Data Registry (4). This report was also typical in that the TG association remained after controlling for total cholesterol levels but was no longer significant after controlling for HDL cholesterol.

To determine if elevations of plasma TG precede the onset of disease, a prospective study design must be used. Many such studies have been conducted in men, with follow-up periods ranging from 3 to 12 years. Although most prospective studies also demonstrate a univariate association between hypertriglyceridemia and CHD (5–7), some investigators found no such association (8,9). The results of multivariate analyses in prospective studies are also much more varied. For example, results from 7-year follow-up in the Western Collaborative Group Study showed a univariate relationship, but this association was no longer significant after adjusting for either LDL cholesterol or HDL cholesterol (5). These results have often been used to argue that TG is not an "independent" risk factor.

In evaluating the role of TG as a risk factor, specific groups of subjects should also be considered. Studies that have performed analyses specific to women have generally found a significant univariate association. In particular, a series of studies in Scandinavia consistently showed that TG correlated strongly with MI but not angina pectoris (6,10). At least four studies that evaluated TG as a risk factor among subjects with normal cholesterol levels have found an association. For example, in the Paris Prospective Study (11), a significant association was found among subjects with total cholesterol less than 220 mg/dl. However, the Rancho Bernardo Study found no such association (9). The role of TG as a risk factor among diabetics and subjects with impaired glucose intolerance has also been considered. In the Paris Prospective Study, a clear relationship was also seen between elevated TG levels and CHD death (12).

Thus, studies in men generally show a univariate association between TG and CHD. In multivariate statistical analyses, this association generally persists after adjustment for total or LDL cholesterol but not after adjustment for HDL cholesterol. In women, normocholesterolemic, and diabetic subjects, TG appears to be a stronger risk factor.

STATISTICAL CONSIDERATIONS

A recent theoretical statistical analysis can help in understanding the apparent discrepancies between the univariate and multivariate results reported in these epidemiologic studies (13). Using simulations based on statistical linear model theory, Davis and Kim set "true" risk ratios for TG ranging from 1.0 to 2.0 and "true" risk ratios for HDL cholesterol ranging from 0.5 to 1.0. Based on previous work, they assumed a strong inverse association between TG and HDL cholesterol, with a correlation coefficient of -0.4. They also assumed both a larger intraindividual variation and a larger interindividual variation for TG compared with HDL cholesterol—also well-documented characteristics. Under these assumptions, they calculated the estimated risk ratio for TG, and compared it with the "true" risk ratio they had set. Over a range of HDL risk ratios, the TG risk ratio was consistently underestimated. For example, for an HDL risk ratio of 0.5 and a true TG risk ratio of 2.0, the estimated risk ratio for TG was 1.60. These results indicate that investigators who use multivariate statistical analyses may underestimate the association of TG and CHD.

GENETIC SUSCEPTIBILITY

Individual genetic susceptibility may also affect the results of the epidemiologic studies described above. For example, Brunzell et al. have shown differential risk of MI in the familial forms of hypertriglyceridemia (14). Familial combined hyperlipidemia (FCHL) is characterized by elevations of plasma cholesterol and/or triglyceride in family members, variable lipoprotein phenotypes, and increased levels of plasma apolipoprotein B. In familial hypertriglyceridemia, only elevations of TG are seen, and the relatives of the patient have cholesterol levels within normal ranges. In a study of 19 families with familial hypertriglyceridemia and 24 families with FCHL, risk of MI among relatives was no greater in familial hypertriglyceridemia than it was in a group of spouse controls. However, the prevalence of MI was nearly double among relatives in families with FCHL (14).

Finally, recent results from our laboratory indicate that there are genetic influences on lipoprotein heterogeneity that are related to TG. Specifically, subclasses of LDL particles have been identified and characterized by size and density (15). Using gradient gel electrophoresis, two distinct LDL subclass patterns denoted patterns A and B, have been identified. LDL subclass pattern A is characterized by a predominance of relatively large, bouyant LDL particles. Approximately 70% of the general population falls into this category. In contrast, LDL subclass pattern B, characterized by a predominance of small, dense LDL particles, is present in about 30% of study subjects (16).

In a study of 61 primarily healthy families, we demonstrated that the inheritance LDL subclass pattern B was consistent with the presence of a single major genetic locus (16). Based on complex segregation analysis, the best genetic model included a dominant mode of inheritance, an allele frequency of 0.25 for the proposed pattern B allele, and reduced penetrance among male subjects under the age of 20 years and premenopausal females. Among the individual family members, a predominance of small, dense LDL was also associated with small but significant increases in adjusted mean LDL cholesterol, decreased HDL cholesterol, and a striking increase in plasma TG (17). Although the lipid values were all within normal ranges, the mean TG value for pattern B subjects was more than 70 mg/dl higher than pattern A subjects.

Based on data from the Boston Area Health Study, a case-control study of MI survivors, we also investigated the association of LDL subclass patterns with risk of MI (18). LDL subclass pattern B was present in 50% of cases but only 26% of controls. The resulting odds ratio was 3.0, a highly significant result ($p < 0.01$). In multivariate statistical analysis, this odds ratios did not decrease after adjustment for LDL cholesterol and was reduced to 2.2 after adjustment for HDL cholesterol ($p < 0.05$). With adjustment for triglyceride, the odds ratio decreased to 1.6 and was no longer significant. However, this result was not surprising, due to the strong association of TG with LDL subclass patterns among both cases and controls. That is, mean levels of TG were significantly higher in subjects with LDL subclass pattern B, regardless of case-control status.

Thus, a predominance of small, dense LDL appears to be a genetically influenced trait that is associated with both increased risk of MI and elevated plasma TG levels.

CONCLUSIONS

Based on the observational epidemiologic evidence, TG is associated with risk of CHD, especially in specific groups of subjects. Although many epidemiologic studies do not suggest that TG has an effect independent of other lipid measures, statistical theory indicates that multivariate statistical analyses underestimate the TG-disease association. Finally, a predominance of small, dense LDL appears to be a marker for a genetic risk of atherosclerosis related to TG.

REFERENCES

1. Albrink MJ, Man EB. Serum triglycerides in coronary artery disease. *Arch Intern Med* 1959;103:4–8.
2. Simons LA. Interrelations of lipids and lipoproteins with coronary artery disease mortality in 19 countries. *Am J Cardiol* 1986;57:5G–10G.
3. Castelli WP, Doyle JT, Gordon T. HDL cholesterol and other lipids in coronary heart disease. The Cooperative Lipoprotein Phenotyping Study. *Circulation* 1977;55:767–772.
4. Freedman DS, Gruchow HW, Anderson AJ, et al. Relation of triglyceride levels to coronary artery disease. The Milwaukee Cardiovascular Data Registry. *Am J Epidemiol* 1988;127:1118–1130.

5. Hulley SB, Rosenman RH, Bawol RD, et al. Epidemiology as a guide to clinical decisions. The association between triglyceride and coronary heart disease. *N Engl J Med* 1980;302:1383–1389.
6. Carlson LA, Bottiger LE. Risk factors for ischaemic heart disease in men and women. Results of the 19-year follow-up of the Stockholm Prospective Study. *Acta Med Scand* 1985;218:207–11.
7. Benfante RJ, Reed DM, MacLean CJ, Yano K. Risk factors in middle age that predict early and late onset of coronary heart disease. *J Clin Epidemiol* 1989;42:95–104.
8. Heyden S, Heiss G, Hames CG, Bartel AG. Fasting triglycerides as predictors of total and CHD mortality in Evans County, Georgia. *J Chronic Dis* 1980;33:275–282.
9. Barrett-Connor E, Khaw K-T. Borderline fasting hypertriglyceridemia. Absence of excess risk of all-cause and cardiovascular disease mortality in healthy men without hypercholesterolemia. *Prev Med* 1987;16:1–8.
10. Lapidus L, Bengtsson C, Lindquist O, Sigurdsson JA, Rybo E. Triglycercides—main lipid risk factor for cardiovascular disease in women? *Acta Med Scand* 1985;217:481–489.
11. Cambien F, Jacqueson A, Richard JL, et al. Is the level of serum triglyceride a significant predictor of coronary death in "normocholesterolemic" subjects? The Paris Prospective Study. *Am J Epidemiol* 1986;124:624–632.
12. Fontbonne E, Eschwege E, Cambien F, et al. Hypertriglyceridemia as a risk factor for coronary heart disease mortality in subjects with impaired glucose tolerance or diabetes. *Diabetologia* 1989;32:300–304.
13. Davis CE, Kim H. Is triglyceride an independent risk factor for CHD? *Circulation* 1990;81:14.
14. Brunzell JD, Schrott HG, Motulsky AG, et al. Myocardial infarction in the familial forms of hypertriglyceridemia. *Metabolism* 1976;25:313–320.
15. Krauss RM, Burke DJ. Identification of multiple subclasses of plasma low density lipoproteins in normal humans. *J Lipid Res* 1982;23:97–104.
16. Austin MA, King M-C, Vranizan KM, Newman B, Krauss RM. Inheritance of low-density lipoprotein subclass patterns: results of complex segregation analysis. *Am J Hum Genet* 1988;43:838–846.
17. Austin MA, King M-C, Vranizan KM, Krauss RM. Atherogenic lipoprotein phenotype: a proposed genetic marker for coronary heart disease risk. *Circulation* 1991;82:495–506.
18. Austin MA, Breslow JL, Hennekens CH, Buring JE, Willett WC, Krauss RM. Low-density lipoprotein subclass patterns and risk of myocardial infarction. *JAMA* 1988;260:1917–1921.

Atherosclerosis Reviews, Volume 22,
edited by A. M. Gotto, Jr. and R. Paoletti.
Raven Press, Ltd., New York © 1991.

The Prognostic Value of Triglycerides in Coronary Heart Disease

Findings from the Helsinki Heart Study

Vesa Manninen, Leena Tenkanen, *Jussi K. Huttunen, and
M. Heikki Frick

*First Department of Medicine, University of Helsinki and *National Public
Health Institute, 00290 Helsinki, Finland*

A major finding of the Helsinki Heart Study (HHS) was that the main fractions of serum cholesterol display high degrees of interdependence as risk factors in coronary heart disease (CHD). Interpretation of the triglyceride (TG) results is less straightforward. This report reviews the main lipid findings from the HHS and presents more detailed analysis of the association between serum TG and the risk of CHD. Are serum TG levels useful in isolation, or does such data only have meaningful predictive value when combined with high-density lipoprotein (HDL) and low-density lipoprotein (LDL) findings?

The design and principle findings of the HHS are described in detail elsewhere (1,2). The HHS was a 5-year, placebo-controlled, double-blind clinical trial designed to test the hypothesis that lowering serum LDL cholesterol and TG levels while elevating serum HDL cholesterol level with the lipid-modulating drug gemfibrozil reduces the incidence of CHD in middle-aged, dyslipidemic men.

SUBJECTS AND METHODS

The participants were selected from 23,531 men aged 40 to 55 years, each employed by one of two state-owned enterprises or five industrial companies in Finland. Volunteers were eligible for the trial if their non–HDL cholesterol—LDL minus very-low-density lipoproteins (VLDL)—exceeded 5.2 mmol/L on two successive occasions and if they had no evidence of CHD. The trial participants were randomly allocated to either gemfibrozil (*n* = 2,046) or placebo (*n* = 2,035).

Cholesterol and TG were measured using enzymatic methods. HDL was determined after precipitation of VLDL and LDL with dextran sulphate–magnesium chloride. The LDL cholesterol concentration was calculated using the formula LDL = total cholesterol minus HDL minus TG divided by 2.2. TG concentrations of ≥ 8.1 mmol/L were excluded from LDL calculations. Computed LDL values < 2.6 mmol/L were also eliminated.

TG values from the second screening visit were taken to represent the pretreatment level of serum TG and were also used for calculating baseline LDL values.

The lipid variables were dichotomized for the analyses as follows: total cholesterol > 7.8 mmol/L, LDL > 5 mmol/L, LDL/HDL > 5, TG > 2 mmol/L. For HDL, we used a cut-off point of < 1.08 mmol/L, which was the lowest tertile in the HHS baseline HDL values.

RESULTS AND DISCUSSION

In the HHS, a 34% reduction in the incidence of definite cardiac endpoints was observed among those receiving gemfibrozil, compared to the men of the placebo group. The reduction became evident during the second year of therapy and grew progressively larger during the following 3 years of the trial.

In the gemfibrozil group, the rise in HDL level was the most significant blood lipid change associated with the reduction in endpoint incidence, although the fall in LDL was also a significant contributor. On the other hand, neither baseline TG nor changes in TG during the trial were significantly associated with risk in the Cox proportional hazards model analysis (2).

In the placebo group, the baseline LDL/HDL cholesterol ratio was the best single lipid predictor of cardiac events. Baseline TG values also showed a significant association with CHD risk, but this relationship vanished when adjusted for HDL. However, a different pattern emerged when the crude incidence data in the placebo group were analyzed by baseline tertiles of TG (≤ 1.4 mmol/L, 1.4-2.1 mmol/L, > 2.1 mmol/L). The highest risk was seen in the highest TG tertile and the lowest risk in the middle tertile.

We then investigated the joint effect of TG and other serum lipids. A cut-off point of 2 mmol/L was chosen to divide men into low and high TG categories. In the placebo group, low TG was associated with low risk in subjects with low and also high serum cholesterol (low ≤ 7.8 mmol/L, high > 7.8 mmol/L). The reduction in endpoints due to gemfibrozil was more pronounced among men with high TG and low total cholesterol, suggesting that both TG and cholesterol levels should be taken into account when gemfibrozil treatment is being considered. The joint effect of TG and LDL (low LDL ≤ 5 mmol/L, high > 5 mmol/L) on CHD incidence in the placebo group showed a similar pattern to that of TG and total cholesterol. Comparison with the treatment group revealed that gemfibrozil was clearly more effective among the low LDL–high TG men than among the high LDL–high TG men. This finding also underscores the prognostic value of combining TG values with other lipid data in risk factor assessment.

HDL levels (low < 1.08 mmol/L, high ≥ 1.08 mmol/L) exerted a considerable influence on the effect of TG on CHD risk. In both categories of HDL, the incidence of CHD among placebo men was > 30% greater when TG was > 2 mmol/L. In the gemfibrozil group, there was a >50% decrease in CHD endpoints among those with low HDL and high TG compared with the placebo group.

The highest risk of CHD in the subgroup analysis was observed in subjects with high LDL/HDL ratio (low ≤ 5, high > 5) and high TG. In the placebo group, the relative risk (RR) of CHD among these subjects was 2.99 (95% confidence interval, 1.75–5.10) compared to those with LDL/HDL ≤ 5 and TG < 2 mmol/L. If TG was > 2 mmol/L and LDL/HDL < 5, the RR was close to unity (0.96). If TG ≤ 2 mmol/L and LDL/HDL > 5, the RR was only 1.11. The group with LDL/HDL > 5 and TG > 2 mmol/L profited most from gemfibrozil treatment. They had a 62% lower risk of CHD than the corresponding placebo subgroup. The treatment effect was small or non-existent in other subgroups formed on the basis of TG and LDL/HDL ratio.

These findings raise questions about the conventional use of regression models; in addition, they may reflect more accurate representations of risks associated with different metabolic states. In other words, it may be inappropriate from the biological viewpoint to be entertaining the possibility of an independent role of TG in the CHD process.

Our findings demonstrate that despite the apparent lack of an independent effect of TG, it is a strong predictor of risk when taken together with LDL (or total) cholesterol and HDL cholesterol. In conclusion, studying the "conditional" effect of TG rather than searching for an independent influence has shown that TG is a useful marker of increased risk of CHD in the Helsinki Heart Study.

REFERENCES

1. Frick MH, Elo O, Haapa K, et al. Helsinki Heart Study: primary prevention trial with gemfibrozil in middle-aged men with dyslipidemia. *N Engl J Med* 1987;317:1237–1245.
2. Manninen V, Elo O, Frick MH, et al. Lipid alterations and decline in the incidence of coronary heart disease in the Helsinki Heart Study. *JAMA* 1988;260:641–651.

Atherosclerosis Reviews, Volume 22,
edited by A. M. Gotto, Jr. and R. Paoletti.
Raven Press, Ltd., New York © 1991.

Triglycerides and Coronary Heart Disease

Michael H. Criqui

*Department of Community and Family Medicine and Department of Medicine,
University of California, San Diego, School of Medicine,
La Jolla, California 92093*

Despite decades of research, and particularly careful scrutiny of this issue in recent years, the status of triglyceride (TG) as an independent risk factor for coronary heart disease (CHD) continues to be controversial (1–4). Various investigations exploring this issue over the last 15 years will be reviewed, including preliminary results from the Lipid Research Clinics Follow-up Study (5).

In case-control studies, TG is routinely found to be a risk factor for various CHD end points. Most studies that have considered myocardial infarction (MI), angina, or coronary disease and adjusted for total or LDL cholesterol, have found that TG represents a persistent independent risk (6–12). Further adjustment for a critical inverse correlate of TG, HDL cholesterol, was reported in only four of these studies (7,10–12). Nevertheless, the association of TG with CHD remained in each of these studies. Investigators looking at the degree of coronary occlusion at angiography consistently report a association with TG even after control for LDL or total cholesterol (13–17). One study controlling for HDL cholesterol reported that the TG association disappeared (17), but another found that the association, prevalent only in women, remained after adjustment for HDL cholesterol (16). Thus, it appears that, despite some contradictory evidence, TG usually retains its status as a risk factor after multivariate adjustment in case-control studies.

Recently, the concept of a pattern B subclass exhibiting an excess of small, dense LDL particles has been introduced. Austin et al. reported that even though cases with nonfatal MI had LDL cholesterol levels similar to controls, they were three times more likely to have pattern B (18). Pattern B is characterized by higher body mass index, higher TG, and lower HDL cholesterol. Interestingly, the authors presented a multivariate analysis of possible explanatory variables for the pattern B effect. TG explained more of the risk of pattern B than any other covariate, including HDL cholesterol; and after adjustment for TG, the original, highly significant relative risk of 3.0 was reduced to 1.6 (p = nonsignificant). In contrast, after adjustment for HDL cholesterol, the relative risk risk was reduced to 2.2 but remained statistically significant.

The limitations of case-control studies are well known. Of particular concern is the fact that the levels of TG or of covariates may have changed since the disease end point. Thus, prospective studies allow stronger etiologic inferences.

Several prospective studies have found TG to be a univariate risk factor, but simultaneous control for total LDL or HDL cholesterol has often reduced the TG association, suggesting that TG is not an independent risk factor (2,19–21). However, seven studies (22–28) have shown TG to be a risk factor independent of cholesterol; in fact, in four of these studies, TG was a stronger risk factor than cholesterol (22–24,28). An additional study found TG to be an independent risk factor for CHD beginning before age 60 but not for CHD with later onset (29). Because none of these studies measured HDL cholesterol, they are subject to criticism. However, the association of TG in previous negative prospective studies was either not present in univariate analysis or was removed after adjustment for only total or LDL cholesterol. In fact, no prospective study has shown a TG association that persisted after adjustment for total or LDL cholesterol but not after adjustment for HDL cholesterol.

There are several important points to keep in mind when investigating TG as a risk factor. First, adjustment for total cholesterol may be inappropriate because in patients with elevated TG, VLDL cholesterol is elevated. Thus, attempting to adjust for LDL cholesterol using total cholesterol may result in overadjustment. Second, TG values are skewed in populations; therefore, either categorical definitions or log transformations should be used. Third, there is a strong inverse correlation between HDL cholesterol and TG; and the lower variability for HDL versus TG may result in overestimating an HDL effect and underestimating a TG effect. A recent computer simulation confirmed this point (30). Finally, certain subgroups, such as women (22,31,32), men with lower total cholesterol (19), or diabetics (33–35), may be particularly susceptible to the effects of TG, so that analysis without special consideration of these subgroups can dilute the association.

In the Lipid Research Clinics (LRC) Follow-up Study, we found a significant association of TG with CHD mortality in men even after adjustment for multiple covariates, including both LDL and HDL cholesterol (5). We avoided adjustment for total cholesterol, and we used log transformation of TG and a categorical definition of high TG. Our study pointed to a slightly greater risk for women than men, even though the rate of actual events was higher in men, and thus, there was more statistical confidence in the estimates. In both men and women with lower HDL and with lower LDL cholesterol, there appeared to be a higher relative risk for TG. In addition, in men, there was evidence for a greater risk of TG at higher levels of fasting plasma glucose. Fasting plasma glucose was a strong CHD risk factor in men, which explained some but not all of the TG association in men. Our results are concordant with earlier suggestions that TG may impart a higher relative risk in persons with low HDL or low LDL, and in diabetics. The relative risks were slightly higher in women than in men in our study. In addition, the concept of a generalized pattern of insulin resistance is suggested by the LRC results, since the subset with low HDL, low to normal LDL, high fasting plasma glucose, and higher body mass index is where TG showed the greatest discriminating power.

Clinical trials have also explored the risk factor status of TG. In the Coronary Drug Project secondary prevention study, niacin resulted in a decrease in CHD mortality and total mortality after 15 years of follow-up in men with MI at baseline (36). However, these men were only under treatment for the first 7 years of the study. The degree of reduction in CHD in the niacin group was related to the degree of cholesterol reduction, but not to the degree of TG lowering. By contrast, in the Stockholm Ischemic Heart Disease Secondary Prevention Study, where survivors of MI were randomized to treatment with clofibrate and niacin or to a control group, reduction in TG was closely correlated with survival, whereas the reduction in cholesterol was not (37). Finally, recent studies of exercise in triathletes and in twins suggest that exercise leads to decreases in triglyceride, increases in HDL cholesterol, and changes toward larger and less dense LDL (38,39).

SUMMARY

A careful review of the literature suggests that the risk factor status of TG is stronger than previously assumed. In addition to being a good univariate marker for increased risk, TG is also an independent risk factor in multivariate analysis. The evidence that TG is a stronger risk factor for certain subsets of the population, such as women, individuals with low LDL, individuals with low HDL, and diabetics, points to a more generalized metabolic condition. The available data indicate that insulin resistance or a related metabolic disorder is likely involved.

However, it is not immediately clear which components of the insulin resistance spectrum are the appropriate targets for clinical intervention. Lipid and lipoprotein levels have been targeted in patients, as has glucose metabolism. Even hypercoaguability, which has been reported to be associated with hypertriglyceridemia (40), may be an important intervention target in this condition. Clearly, we need intensive investigation to uncover the mechanism by which TG is related to CHD. In the interim, while various behavioral and pharmacologic therapies are being evaluated, we can take comfort in knowing that physical activity exerts a favorable influence on the abnormalities associated with the insulin resistance syndrome and that both weight loss and improved diet should also mitigate this condition.

ACKNOWLEDGMENTS

Dr. Criqui is the recipient of a Preventive Cardiology Academic Award (HL 01718-03) from the National Institutes of Health, National Heart, Lung and Blood Institute.

REFERENCES

1. Austin MA. Plasma triglyceride as a risk factor for coronary heart disease: the epidemiologic evidence and beyond. *Am J Epidemiol* 1989;129:249.
2. Hulley SB, et al. Epidemiology as a guide to clinical decisions: the association between triglyceride and coronary heart disease. *N Engl J Med* 1980;302:1383.
3. Nestel PJ. Is serum triglyceride an independent predictor of coronary artery disease? *Pract Cardiol* 1987;13:96.
4. Avins AL, Haber RJ, Hulley SB. The status of hypertriglyceridemia as a risk factor for coronary heart disease. *Clin Lab Med* 1989;9:153.
5. Criqui MH, et al. Triglycerides and coronary heart disease mortality: the Lipid Research Clinics follow-up study [Abstract]. *Cardio Vasc Dis Epidemiol Newsletter* 1987;41:13.
6. Brunner D, et al. Serum cholesterol and triglyceride in patients suffering for ischemic heart disease and in healthy subjects. *Atherosclerosis* 1977;28:197.
7. Castelli WP, et al. HDL cholesterol and other lipids in coronary heart disease. The Co-operative Lipoprotein Phenotyping Study. *Circulation* 1977;55:767.
8. Wilhelmsen L, et al. Multiple risk prediction of myocardial infarction in women as compared with men. *Br Heart J* 1977;39:1179.
9. Scott DW, Gotto AM, Cole JS, Gorry GA. Plasma lipids as collateral risk factors in coronary artery disease: a study of 371 males with chest pain. *J Chronic Dis* 1978;31:337.
10. Fager G, et al. Multivariate analyses of serum apolipoproteins and risk factors in relation to acute myocardial infarction. *Arteriosclerosis* 1981;1:273.
11. Kukita H, et al. Plasma lipids and lipoproteins in Japanese male patients with coronary artery disease and in their relatives. *Atherosclerosis* 1982;42:21.
12. Hamsten A, et al. Serum lipoproteins and apolipoproteins in young male survivors of myocardial infarction. *Atherosclerosis* 1986;59:223.
13. Gotto AM, et al. Relationship between plasma lipid concentrations and coronary artery disease in 496 patients. *Circulation* 1977;56:875.
14. Anderson AJ, Barboriak JJ, Rimm AA. Risk factors in angiographically determined coronary occlusion. *Am J Epidemiol* 1978;107:8.
15. Cabin HS, Roberts WC. Relation of serum total cholesterol and triglyceride levels to the amount and extent of coronary arterial narrowing by atherosclerotic plaque in coronary heart disease: quantitative analysis of 2,037 five mm segments of 160 major epicardial coronary arteries in 40 necropsy patients. *Am J Med* 1982;73:227.
16. Reardon MF, et al. Lipoprotein predictors of the severity of coronary artery disease in men and women. *Circulation* 1985;71:881.
17. Freedman DS, et al. Relation of triglyceride levels to coronary disease: the Milwaukee Cardiovascular Data Registry. *Am J Epidemiol* 1988;127:1118.
18. Austin MA, et al. Low-density lipoprotein subclass patterns and risk of myocardial infarction. *JAMA* 1988;260:1917.
19. Cambien F, et al. Is the level of serum triglyceride a significant predictor of coronary death in "normocholesterolemic" subjects? *Am J Epidemiol* 1986;124:624.
20. Salonen J, Puska P. Relation of serum cholesterol and triglycerides to the risk of acute myocardial infarction, cerebral stroke and death in eastern Finnish male population. *Int J Epidemiol* 1983;12:26.
21. Pocock SJ, Shaper AG, Phillips AN. Concentrations of high density lipoprotein cholesterol, triglycerides, and total cholesterol in ischaemic heart disease. *Br Med J* 1989;298:998.
22. Lapidus L, et al. Triglycerides—main lipid risk factor for cardiovascular disease in women? *Acta Med Scand* 1985;217:481.

23. Petersson B, Trell E, Hood B. Premature death and associated risk factors in urban middle-aged men. *Am J Med* 1984;77:418.
24. Carlson LA, Böttiger LE. Risk factors for ischemic heart disease in men and women: results of the 19-year follow-up of the Stockholm Prospective Study. *Acta Med Scand* 1985;218:207.
25. Åberg H, et al. Serum triglycerides are a risk factor for myocardial infarction but not for angina pectoris. *Atherosclerosis* 1985;54:89.
26. Pelkonen R, et al. Association of serum lipids and obesity with cardiovascular mortality. *Br Med J* 1977;2:1185.
27. Tverdal A, et al. Serum triglycerides as an independent risk factor for death from coronary heart disease in middle-aged Norwegian men. *Am J Epidemiol* 1989;129:458.
28. Glynn RJ, Rosner B, Silber JE. Changes in cholesterol and triglyceride as predictors of ischemic heart disease in men. *Circulation* 1982;66:724.
29. Benfante RJ, et al. Risk factors in middle age that predict early and late onset of coronary heart disease. *J Clin Epidemiol* 1989;42:95.
30. Davis CE, Kim H. Is triglyceride level an independent risk factor for CHD? [Abstract]. *Circulation* 1990;81:725.
31. Heyden S, et al. Fasting triglycerides as predictors of total and CHD mortality in Evans County, Georgia. *J Chronic Dis* 1980;33:275.
32. Castelli WP. The triglyceride issue: a view from Framingham. *Am Heart J* 1986;112:432.
33. Fontbonne A, et al. Hypertriglyceridaemia as a risk factor of coronary heart disease mortality in subjects with impaired glucose tolerance or diabetes: results from the 11-year follow-up of the Paris Prospective Study. *Diabetologia* 1989;32:300.
34. West KM, et al. The role of circulating glucose and triglyceride concentrations and their interactions with other "risk factors" as determinants of arterial disease in nine diabetic population samples from the WHO Multinational Study. *Diabetes Care* 1983;6:361.
35. Janka HU. Five-year incidence of major microvascular complications in diabetes mellitus. *Horm Metabol Res[Suppl]* 1985;15:15.
36. Canner PL, et al. Fifteen year mortality in coronary drug project patients. Long-term benefit with niacin. *J Am Coll Cardiol* 1986;8:1245.
37. Carlson LA, Rosenhamer G. Reduction of mortality in the Stockholm Ischaemic Heart Disease Secondary Prevention Study by combined treatment with clofibrate and nicotinic acid. *Acta Med Scand* 1988;223:405.
38. Lamon-Fava S, et al. Changes in lipids, apolipoproteins, and low density lipoprotein particle size after prolonged strenuous physical exercise [Abstract]. *Clin Res* 1988;36:787.
39. Wu LL, et al. Genetic concordance of and exercise effects on low density lipoprotein subfractions in Utah twins [Abstract]. *Circulation* 1988;78(suppl II):II-481.
40. Simpson HCR, et al. Hypertriglyceridemia and hypercoaguability. *Lancet* 1983;1:786.

Atherosclerosis Reviews, Volume 22,
edited by A. M. Gotto, Jr. and R. Paoletti.
Raven Press, Ltd., New York © 1991.

Hypertriglyceridemia, Triglyceride-Rich Lipoproteins, and Coronary Atherosclerosis

Anders Hamsten, Per Tornvall, Jan Johansson,
Fredrik Karpe, and Lars A. Carlson

King Gustaf V Research Institute and Department of Internal Medicine,
Karolinska Hospital, Karolinska Institute, S-10401 Stockholm, Sweden

The relationships among hypertriglyceridemia, triglyceride-rich lipoproteins (TGRLP), and coronary atherosclerosis remain obscure. In the past few years, however, detailed metabolic and cell biological studies have suggested that there are direct mechanisms whereby TGRLP might be implicated in atherogenesis. The hypertriglyceridemic state has also been shown to act indirectly on the processes leading to atherosclerosis by influencing the metabolism and composition of intermediate-density lipoprotein (IDL), low-density lipoprotein (LDL), and high-density lipoprotein (HDL). There is also an abundance of data suggesting that hypertriglyceridemic subjects have delayed clearance of postprandial lipoproteins, which may be taken up by arterial wall macrophages.

This brief review aims at presenting the evidence that TGRLP are major factors in the processes leading to premature coronary atherosclerosis; it further attempts to delineate the mechanisms by which these actions are exerted.

DIRECT EFFECTS OF VERY LOW DENSITY LIPOPROTEINS AND THEIR REMNANTS

Whether very-low-density lipoproteins (VLDL) are atherogenic may depend in part on their ability to penetrate into the subintimal layers of the arterial wall. Normally, the larger VLDL particles do not pass the endothelial barrier. However, the presence of endothelial injury may facilitate the passage of even the large VLDL species. Furthermore, most of the circulating VLDL are partially catabolized VLDL particles, commonly referred to as VLDL remnants. The VLDL particles present in hypertriglyceridemia are probably more atherogenic than normolipidemic VLDL, as they have increased affinity to B,E receptors (1,2). Indeed, there is experimental evidence that all hypertriglyceridemic VLDL particles, but only very small (S_f 20–60) normolipidemic VLDL will bind to the B,E receptor. The apolipoprotein B (apoB) molecules contained in TGRLP of certain hypertriglyceridemic subjects may may also become partially degraded. This alteration could promote binding to an unregulated macrophage receptor, which is distinct from the B,E receptor (3).

DETERMINATION OF LDL HETEROGENEITY

To a large extent, the plasma VLDL level determines the particle size distribution, density, and chemical composition of LDL by promoting exchange of triglyceride (TG) from VLDL for cholesteryl ester from LDL through lipid transfer proteins (4). TG-enriched LDL particles formed during the lipid transfer reaction in hypertriglyceridemia subsequently undergo a continuous size reduction through the action of lipases, which results in protein-rich and lipid-poor particles of higher density. Although small, protein-enriched LDL particles make up a larger proportion of the total LDL population in patients with coronary heart disease (CHD), it is far from obvious that these particles per se are atherogenic. Circumstances associated with the formation of dense LDL, such as overproduction of VLDL apoB and slow LDL catabolism, may represent the direct atherogenic mechanism. If so, LDL heterogeneity would constitute an epiphenomenon. Not least because the VLDL TG concentration is associated with a dense LDL pattern, it could be inferred that disturbances in the metabolism of TGRLP represent the underlying pathogenic mechanism. Thus, the increased plasma levels of dense LDL in subjects with premature CHD primarily reflect enhanced transfer of cholesteryl esters to large VLDL for subsequent elimination from the plasma compartment into macrophages and through the B,E receptor.

Compositional changes in plasma LDL induced by lipid transfer proteins might also result in alterations in the cellular metabolism of the modified LDL itself. Hypertriglyceridemic LDL has been shown to exhibit lower affinity toward the B,E receptor in cultured human fibroblasts and to be a less efficient regulator of cellular sterol synthesis and receptor activity (5). Furthermore, normalization of the core lipid composition of hypertriglyceridemic LDL results in conformational changes of the apoB moiety of the particles and nearly normal cellular processing (6).

INFLUENCE ON HDL METABOLISM AND REVERSE CHOLESTEROL TRANSPORT

Close metabolic connections between VLDL and HDL involve extensive exchange of lipid and apolipoprotein constituents between the two systems.

Consequently, disturbances of VLDL metabolism directly influence HDL composition and subclass distribution in plasma. It is still unclear whether these interrelations account for any direct atherogenic effects of VLDL or distort reverse cholesterol transport by HDL.

In a recent angiographic study, plasma HDL subclass levels determined by gradient gel electrophoresis were related to global severity and rate of progression of coronary atherosclerosis (7). Highly significant inverse correlations were found between the concentrations of the largest HDL particles, the HDL_{2b} subclass, and both disease severity and progression over time. However, by analyzing the patients according to lipoprotein phenotype, we observed that the negative relationship between plasma HDL_{2b} concentration and coronary atherosclerosis was only present in normotriglyceridemic subjects who generally had HDL_{2b} values within the normal range. In contrast, the smaller HDL species, HDL_{3b}, had a positive association with progression of coronary atherosclerosis in the hypertriglyceridemic patients, in whom this subclass was elevated. Accordingly, the hypertriglyceridemic state appeared to markedly influence the relations between plasma concentrations of HDL subclasses and coronary atherosclerosis.

Lipid transfer and hepatic lipase activities, in particular, are likely to affect the relations between HDL subspecies and coronary atherosclerosis in hypertriglyceridemic subjects. The higher HDL_{2b} concentration in normo- compared with young hypertriglyceridemic postinfarction patients can thus most likely be explained by less TG transfer to HDL and reduced conversion of HDL_{2b} to HDL_3. In contrast, both the deficiency of HDL_2 and the small particle size of HDL_3 in subjects with hypertriglyceridemia (7a) are probably the consequence of the sequential actions of lipid transfer protein and hepatic lipase on HDL, as indicated by extensive *in vitro* studies (8).

GENERATION OF ATHEROGENIC POSTPRANDIAL LIPOPROTEINS

The question of whether postprandial lipoproteins are atherogenic has not been finally settled, not least because of the paucity of clinical studies in subjects with premature coronary atherosclerosis. Several experimental studies have demonstrated that uptake of chylomicron remnants by macrophages may lead to intracellular accumulation of cholesteryl esters and conversion into foam cells. If chylomicron remnants are atherogenic in man, then delayed removal of these particles might contribute to development of CHD, particularly in hypertriglyceridemic subjects. Evidence of chylomicron remnant retention has been obtained in several studies of hypertriglyceridemic patients (9). TGRLP from both the liver and the intestine make a significant contribution to postprandial triglyceridemia (10). The question thus arises whether elevated plasma levels of chylomicron or VLDL remnants, or both, convert the postalimentary period into an atherogenic state.

During alimentary lipemia, there is pronounced stimulation of cholesteryl ester transfer (11). Accordingly, hypertriglyceridemic subjects with low HDL cholesterol concentration might have accelerated transfer of cholesteryl esters into TGRLP during alimentary lipemia, which contributes to cholesteryl ester accumulation in atherogenic apoB-containing lipoproteins. Patsch et al. (12,13) have also linked the chylomicron remnant hypothesis to the known inverse relationship between HDL and CHD. According to their concept, individuals with normal fasting plasma lipids and high levels of HDL_2 catabolize chylomicrons and chylomicron remnants at a faster rate than individuals with normal fasting lipids and low HDL_2. High plasma concentrations of HDL_2 are consequently considered to be a result rather than a cause of processes that protect against atherosclerosis, as discussed in the previous section.

IMPAIRED FIBRINOLYTIC FUNCTION

Of all hemostatic disturbances associated with thrombotic disease known to date, impaired fibrinolytic function is by far the most commonly observed abnormality. Numerous cross-sectional studies of patients with angina pectoris or previous myocardial infarction (MI) have shown a decreased fibrinolytic activity in patients compared with controls (14). The major mechanism for the fibrinolytic impairment seen in patients with CHD is beyond doubt plasminogen activator inhibitor type 1 activity (PAI-1) elevation in plasma. The positive and fairly strong relationship between serum triglycerides and PAI-1 levels in plasma (15) is of particular interest, because it raises the possibility that hypertriglyceridemia is connected with a predisposition to thrombosis through a coexisting increase in PAI-1 concentration. At present, there is no firm evidence from clinical studies in humans that fibrinolysis plays a significant part in atherogenesis.

The physiological mechanisms regulating PAI-1 secretion from various cells to plasma are poorly established. Alessi et al. (16) recently showed that insulin induces a dose-dependent increase of the PAI-1 secretion by Hep G2 cells in culture, whereas no effect of insulin in this respect was obtained on human umbilical vein endothelial cells. Against this background, we considered it of interest to investigate the relationships of VLDL and LDL to release of PAI-1 from endothelial cells (17). Our results indicate that VLDL stimulates PAI-1 secretion and that hypertriglyceridemic VLDL is a more potent stimulus than normotriglyceridemic VLDL. The mechanism underlying this effect involves binding of VLDL to the B,E receptor, which is more effective in hypertriglyceridemia.

SYNDROME X

The clustering of hypertriglyceridemia with low HDL, hypertension, abdominal obesity, and insulin resistance—a syndrome termed "syndrome X"—and the association of hyperinsulinemia with jointly disturbed plasma VLDL, LDL, and HDL levels (18) have gained considerable attention in the past few years. Insulin resistance is generally accepted as the basic pathogenic mechanism underlying these multiple metabolic disturbances. Given that premise, the resulting hyperinsulinemia is either directly implicated in atherogenesis (19) or acts indirectly through its effects on VLDL metabolism and through stimulation of synthesis and secretion of free PAI-1 from hepatocytes. Thus, insulin could be an intermediate risk factor for CHD that exerts many of its effects through modification of other risk factors, including TGRLP.

CONCLUSIONS

The failure of most epidemiological studies to demonstrate an independent statistical association between hypertriglyceridemia and future CHD should not be taken to rule out the hypertriglyceridemic state or TGRLP themselves as important factors in the processes that lead to coronary atherosclerosis and promote coronary thrombosis. Hypertriglyceridemia has profound effects on the composition of all plasma lipoproteins and on their function in cell biological systems and most likely increases their atherogenicity.

ACKNOWLEDGMENTS

Support for this work was provided by the Swedish Medical Research Council (grants 204 and 08691) and the Swedish Heart-Lung Foundation. Dr. Hamsten is the recipient of a grant from the Swedish Medical Research Council (19P-08152).

REFERENCES

1. Gianturco SH, Gotto AM Jr, Hwang S-LC, et al. Apolipoprotein E mediates uptake of Sf 100–400 hypertriglyceridemic very low density lipoproteins by the low density lipoprotein receptor pathway in normal human fibroblasts. *J Biol Chem* 1983;258:4526–4533.
2. Bradley WA, Hwang S-LC, Karlin JB, et al. Low-density lipoprotein receptor binding determinants switch from apolipoprotein E to apolipoprotein B during conversion of hypertriglyceridemic very-low density lipoprotein to low-density lipoproteins. *J Biol Chem* 1984;259:14728–14735.
3. Gianturco SH, Lin AH-Y, Hwang S-LC, et al. Distinct murine macrophage receptor pathway for human triglyceride-rich lipoproteins. *J Clin Invest* 1988;82:1633–1643.
4. Deckelbaum RJ, Granot E, Oschry Y, Rose L, Eisenberg S. Plasma triglyceride determines

structure-composition in low and high density lipoproteins. *Arteriosclerosis* 1984;4:225–231.

5. Kleinman Y, Eisenberg S, Oschry Y, Gavish D, Stein O, Stein Y. Defective metabolism of hypertriglyceridemic low density lipoprotein in cultured human skin fibroblasts. *J Clin Invest* 1985;75:1796–1803.

6. Kleinman Y, Schonfeld G, Gavish D, Oschry Y, Eisenberg S. Hypolipidemic therapy modulates expression of apolipoprotein B epitopes on low density lipoproteins. Studies in mild to moderate hypertriglyceridemic patients. *J Lipid Res* 1987;28:540–548.

7. Johansson J, Carlson LA, Landou C, Hamsten A. High density lipoproteins and coronary atherosclerosis. A strong inverse relation with the largest particles is confined to normotriglyceridemic patients. *Atherosclerosis Thromb* 1991;11:174–182.

7a.Chang LBF, Hopkins GJ, Barter PJ. Particle size distribution of high density lipoproteins as a function of plasma triglyceride concentration in human subjects. *Atherosclerosis* 1985;56:61–70.

8. Hopkins GJ, Barter PJ. Role of triglyceride-rich lipoproteins and hepatic lipase in determining the particle size and compositions of high density lipoproteins. *J Lipid Res* 1986;27:1265–1277.

9. Wilson DE, Chan I-F, Buchi KN, Horton SC. Postchallenge plasma lipoprotein retinoids: chylomicron remnants in endogenous hypertriglyceridemia. *Metabolism* 1985;34:551–558.

10. Cohn JS, McNamara JR, Cohn SD, Ordovas JM, Schaefer EJ. Plasma apolipoprotein changes in the triglyceride-rich lipoprotein fraction of human subjects fed a fat-rich meal. *J Lipid Res* 1988;29:925–936.

11. Tall A, Sammett D, Granot E. Mechanisms of enhanced cholesteryl ester transfer from high density lipoproteins to apolipoprotein B–containing lipoproteins during alimentary lipemia. *J Clin Invest* 1986;77:1163–1172.

12. Patsch JR, Karlin JB, Scott LW, Smith LC, Gotto Jr AM. Inverse relationship between blood levels of high density lipoprotein subfraction 2 and magnitude of postprandial lipemia. *Proc Nat Acad Sci USA* 1983;80:1449–1453.

13. Patsch JR, Prasad S, Gotto AM Jr, Bengtsson-Olivecrona G. Postprandial lipemia. A key for the conversion of high density lipoprotein2 into high density lipoprotein3 by hepatic lipase. *J Clin Invest* 1984;74:2017–2023.

14. Wiman B, Hamsten A. The fibrinolytic enzyme system and its role in the etiology of thrombotic disease. *Semin Thromb Hemost* 1990;16:207–216.

15. Hamsten A, Wiman B, de Faire U, Blombäck M. Increased plasma levels of a rapid inhibitor of tissue plasminogen activator in young survivors of myocardial infarction. *N Engl J Med* 1985;313:1557–1563.

16. Alessi MC, Juhan-Vague I, Kooistra T, Declerck PJ, Collen D. Insulin stimulates the synthesis of plasminogen activator inhibitor 1 by the human hepatocellular cell line Hep G2. *Thromb Haemost* 1988;60:491–494.

17. Stiko-Rahm A, Wiman B, Hamsten A, Nilsson J. Secretion of plasminogen activator inhibitor from cultured human umbilical vein endothelial cells is induced by very low density lipoprotein. *Arteriosclerosis* 1990;10:1067–1073.

18. Modan M, Halkin H, Lusky A, Segal P, Fuchs Z, Chetrit A. Hyperinsulinemia is characterized by jointly disturbed plasma VLDL, LDL, and HDL levels. A population-based study. *Arteriosclerosis* 1988;8:227–236.

19. Stout RW. Insulin and atheroma—an update. *Lancet* 1987;1:1077–1079

Atherosclerosis Reviews, Volume 22,
edited by A. M. Gotto, Jr. and R. Paoletti.
Raven Press, Ltd., New York © 1991.

Plasma Triglyceride-Rich Lipoproteins and Peripheral Atherosclerosis

Anders G. Olsson, Uno Erikson, Jörgen Mölgaard, and
Gunnar Ruhn

*Department of Internal Medicine, Faculty of Health Sciences, Linköping
University, and Department of Diagnostic Radiology, University Hospital,
Uppsala, Sweden*

In a study of markedly hyperlipidemic but asymtomatic patients, early signs of peripheral artery disease (PAD) were found in patients with types IIB, III, and IV hyperlipoproteinemia (HLP) (1), especially if they were smokers and over 50 years of age (2). Abnormal peripheral circulation was thus found in types of HLP with elevated triglyceride-rich, very-low-density lipoproteins.

There are a number of reasons why subclinical peripheral atherosclerosis provides an excellent model for therapeutic approaches. First, regression of atherosclerosis is probably easier to achieve in an early stage of the disease. Second, the methodology for atheroma quantitation is less complicated in PAD than in coronary atherosclerosis.

Therefore, we decided to perform arteriographies of the femoral arteries with the ultimate goal of achieving a reproducible quantitation of femoral atheroma volume. To do this, automatic techniques are desirable, including microdensitometry and computer estimation of atheroma volume (3,4). In the present study however, results made by visual estimation were assessed by an expert panel.

MATERIALS AND METHODS

From a health-control study of approximately 20,000 randomly selected individuals, all persons with markedly elevated plasma cholesterol (> 9.5 mmol/L) or triglyceride (TG) (> 3.5 mmol/l) who were free from cardiovascular disease were recruited for further investigation and treatment (5). Of this group, 18 type IIA, 18 type IIB, and 24 type IV men were investigated with femoral arteriography (6). Femoral atherosclerosis was estimated by an expert panel whose members were unaware of the clinical and laboratory status of the patients. The femoral artery was divided into four segments, and each segment was evaluated according to the following scoring system:

0 = no visible atherosclerosis
1 = single plaque < 50% of vessel diameter
2 = more than one plaque < 50% of vessel diameter
3 = single plaque > 50% of vessel diameter
4 = more than one plaque > 50% of vessel diameter
5 = complete occlusion

An overall atherosclerosis score (OAS) was created by dividing the sum of segment scores by the number of judged segments. This score served as one measure of femoral atheroma change over time. It was also assessed by direct visual comparison of pairs of angiograms before and after 12 months of treatment.

After receiving dietary treatment for 6 months, subjects who showed femoral atherosclerosis were allocated to either a treatment group with plasma lipid–lowering drug therapy (drug treatment consisted of nicotinic acid 1 g four times daily plus fenofibrate 0.2 g twice daily) or to continued dietary plus placebo treatment. Femoral arteriography was repeated immediately before allocation to treatment group and after 12 months of treatment (7). The radiologic expert panel was unaware of which treatment the patient had received. In addition, quantitative plasma lipoprotein analysis was performed every 2nd month during the study (8).

RESULTS

Prevalence of Femoral Atherosclerosis

Femoral atherosclerosis was found in 13 of 18 (72%), 14 of 18 (78%), and 18 of 24 (75%) cases in types IIA, IIB, and IV HLP, respectively (9). The mean OAS values in patients with atherosclerosis in the corresponding types were 0.58, 0.75, and 0.49, respectively. Atherosclerosis was most severe in type IIB subjects. In all types, atherosclerosis increased as the segment became more distal. Univariate analysis showed that low-density lipoprotein (LDL) cholesterol was significantly related to PAD.

Effect of Treatment on Atheroma Development

The effect of treatment on plasma lipoprotein concentrations is shown in Fig. 1–3 (10). Significant pronounced and sustained decreases were achieved in plasma very-low-density lipoprotein (VLDL) and LDL concentrations, whereas high-density lipoprotein (HDL) increased markedly.

The effect of treatment on atheroma development using the OAS scoring

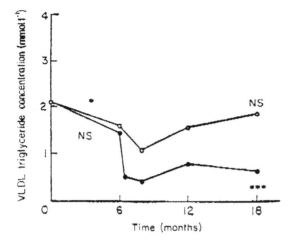

FIG. 1. Changes in VLDL triglyceride concentration in the treatment and control groups during the 18-month study period. Filled circles indicate the treatment group and unfilled circles indicate the control group. Statistical changes are marked on the left for 0–6 months and on the right for 6–18 months, both for the treatment and control group. NS = not significant, i.e., $p > 0.05$. * $= 0.01 < p < 0.05$, ***$p < 0.001$.

method is shown in Table 1 (7). Although the proportion of subjects showing progression was equal in the two groups—about 20%—regression occurred only in the treatment group. Thus, there were fewer cases of unchanged atherosclerosis in the treatment group. The difference in distribution was highly significant. Using the intrapair comparing method, we found the same significant result—i.e., regression only in the treatment group.

Multiple regression analysis was performed to elucidate the role of risk factors and plasma lipoproteins on atherosclerosis outcome. Decreases in systolic blood pressure and plasma VLDL cholesterol related significantly and independently to regression of femoral atherosclerosis.

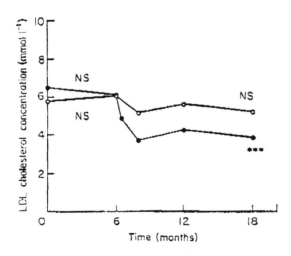

FIG. 2. Changes in LDL cholesterol concentration in the treatment and control groups during the 18-month study period.

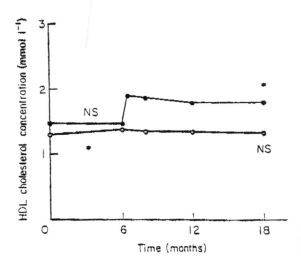

FIG. 3. Changes in HDL cholesterol concentration in the treatment and control groups during the 18-month study period.

DISCUSSION

This 1-year study of asymptomatic hyperlipidemic subjects showed regression of femoral atherosclerosis in almost half (47%) of the cases after strenuous plasma lipid regulation. Regression was related to decreases in triglyceride-rich lipoproteins (TGRLP) and systolic blood pressure, the latter in spite of the fact that all subjects were normotensive.

Ours is not the first study to describe early changes in peripheral arteries after lipid lowering treatment. In 1970, Zelis et al. (10) reported improvement of the diminished peak reactive hyperemia blood flow in type III HLP after treatment with diet and clofibrate for only 3–6 months. In an uncontrolled study of 25 patients with type II and IV HLP, most of them asymptomatic, who were treated with diet plus clofibrate and/or neomycin, Barndt et al. (11) found that nine (36%) showed regression after a mean interval of 13 months. The time interval and proportion of regression thus were similar to our results. Those cases showing regression had significant declines in plasma cholesterol, TG, and blood pressure, findings that also are in agreement with the present study.

TABLE 1. *Changes in OAS after 12 months between treatment and control groups*

	Progression	Unchanged	Regression
Treatment ($n = 17$)[a]	3 (18%)	6 (35%)	8 (47%)
Control	5 (20%)	20 (80%)	0

[a] Eighteen-month angiogram not performed in three cases. Distribution difference $p < 0.001$.

The mechanism behind the regression in the treatment group is most probable through the pronounced effect of lowering atherogenic lipoproteins, particularly the TG-rich fraction of apolipoprotein B–containing ones. This conclusion is in line with current knowledge of risk factors for peripheral atherosclerosis, a condition in which plasma TG are often elevated (11,12).

However, other mechanisms behind the effects observed on atheroma development also deserve consideration. Could nicotinic acid influence blood pressure and myocardial workload, thereby changing the angiograms to simulate regression? The relations between decrease in systolic blood pressure and regression support this interpretation. However, we do not believe this to be true. First, the same relation was found by Barndt et al., but they did not use nicotinic acid (11). Second, the vast majority of the patients were normotensive and free from cardiac disease, which should minimize any central cardiovascular effect by nicotinic acid.

In conclusion, 1 year of intense plasma lipid regulatory treatment can reverse the atheromatous process of the femoral artery in up to 50% of asymtomatic cases. The factors related to the response are TGRLP and blood pressure.

ACKNOWLEDGMENTS

This work was supported by grants from the Swedish Medical Research Council (19M-06962).

REFERENCES

1. Beaumont JL, Carlson LA, Cooper GR, et al. Classification of hyperlipoproteinaemias. *Bull WHO* 1970;43:891.
2. Olsson AG, Eklund B. Studies in asymptomatic primary hyperlipidaemia. V. Peripheral circulation. *Acta Med Scand* 1975;198:197–206.
3. Crawford DW, Brooks SH, Selzer RH, et al. Computer densitometry for angiographic assessment of arterial cholesterol content and gross pathology in human atherosclerosis. *J Lab Clin Med* 1977;89:378–392.
4. Nilsson S, Berglund I, Bylund H, et al. Quantitation of atherosclerosis in femoral arteriography with ECG gated exposures. *Acta Radiol* 1988;29:311.
5. Olsson AG, Carlson LA. Studies in asymptomatic primary hyperlipidaemia. I. Types of hyperlipoproteinaemias and serum lipoprotein concentrations, compositions and interrelations. *Acta Med Scand* 1975;suppl 580:1.
6. Erikson U, Helmius G, Hemmingsson A, Ruhn G, Olsson AG. Repeat femoral arteriography in hyperlipidemic patients. *Acta Radiol Diagn* 1988;29:303–309.
7. Olsson AG, Ruhn G, Erikson U. The effect of serum lipid regulation on the development of femoral atherosclerosis in hyperlipidaemia. A nonrandomized controlled study. *J Intern Med* 1990;227:381–390.
8. Carlson K. Lipoprotein fractionation. *J Clin Pathol* 1973;26 (suppl 5):32–37.
9. Ruhn G, Erikson U, Olsson AG. Prevalence of femoral atherosclerosis in asymptomatic men with hyperlipoproteinaemia *J Intern Med* 1989;225:317–323
10. Zelis R, Mason DT, Braunwald E, Levy RI. Effects of hyperlipoproteinemias and their treatment on the peripheral circulation. *J Clin Invest* 1970;49:1007–1011.

11. Barndt R, Blankenhorn DH, Crawford DW, Brooks SH. Regression and progression of early femoral atherosclerosis in treated hyperlipoproteinemic patients. *Ann Intern Med* 1977;86:139–146.
12. Mölgaard J, von Schenck H, Olsson A. Plasmalipoproteiner och apolipoproteiner hos slumvist utvalda män med claudicatio intermittens. *Svenshaläkaresällskapets Handlingan* 1989;98:183–184.

Atherosclerosis Reviews, Volume 22,
edited by A. M. Gotto, Jr. and R. Paoletti.
Raven Press, Ltd., New York © 1991.

The Low High-Density Lipoprotein/Hypertriglyceridemia Syndrome as a Genetic Risk

A Factor for Coronary Atherosclerosis

D. J. Galton

Medical Unit, St. Bartholomew's Hospital, London EC1A.7BE, England

Recent studies have shown that one of the commonest lipid abnormalities associated with premature coronary artery disease (CAD) is hypertriglyceridaemia with low high-density lipoprotein (HDL) (1,2). In one study of 101 pedigrees, 14.5% of the subjects had this syndrome, whereas 5% had familial combined hyperlipidemia and 1% had familial hypercholesterolemia (1). The genetic determinants underlying these lipid phenotypes may relate to the rare monogenic diseases that produce the uncommon forms of hyperlipidemia. For example, rare mutants of lipoprotein lipase or apolipoprotein C-II (apoC-II) can produce an inherited hypertriglyceridemia. It is possible that commoner disease-related alleles at this locus are responsible for the incidence of this lipid abnormality in the general population.

THE ApoA-I/C-III/A-IV GENE CLUSTER

Many previous studies have implicated mutations at the apoA-I/C-III/A-IV gene cluster on chromosome 11 as contributors to the heritability of hypertriglyceridemia with low HDL (3) or the development of premature atherosclerosis (4,5). For example, a C to G substitution in exon 4 of the apoC-III gene was found at increased frequency in survivors of myocardial infarction (MI) (0.03 controls, $n = 136$; 0.20 patients, $n = 56$, $p < 0.05$), as well as in patients with proven coronary atherosclerosis by angiography (0.03 controls, $n = 136$; 0.11 patients, $n = 121$, $p < 0.01$). More recent studies have confirmed this observation. In one study, the rarer alleles at four polymorphic loci at the A-I/C-III/A-IV gene cluster was found at increased frequency in patients with coronary artery disease with a positive family history compared to subjects with no family history of the disease (6).

These polymorphic sites are probably acting as linkage markers for an etiological mutation in the vicinity. Two possible mechanisms have been postulated. One is an effect on mRNA stability that impairs the induction of these apolipoproteins after a dietary load of fat. The other is possible linkage to promoter mutations in the 5'-regulatory sequences of these apolipoproteins. One mutation that has been studied recently is a G to A substitution at position -78 in the apoA-I promoter. Studies on the frequencies of these alternative alleles have shown differences between the upper and lower deciles for the HDL cholesterol distribution in the general population; this may affect the synthesis of apoA-I for HDL production. *In vitro* transcriptional assays are needed to clarify the role of this promoter mutation in the regulation of apoA-I gene expression.

THE LIPOPROTEIN LIPASE GENE

The gene for human lipoprotein lipase has been recently cloned and localized to chromosome 8. It contains the exons coding for a protein of 65,000 kDa (7). Two common polymorphisms have been observed with the enzymes Hind III and Pvu II; the former is approximately 1.7 kb downstream from exon 10, and the latter is within intron 6. The rare allele at Hind III site shows strong associations with hypertriglyceridemia/low HDL (H2 allele, 0.58 controls, $n = 186$; 0.79 patients, $n = 90$, $p < 0.01$). The differences are also observed in premature coronary atherosclerosis (H2 allele, 0.57 controls, $n = 196$; 0.77 patients, $n = 126$, $p < 0.001$). This makes the locus a likely candidate for one of the genetic determinants of premature coronary atherosclerosis (8). This matter requires further study, with particular attention to exon mutations in the vicinity of the Hind III site.

A summary of the relative strengths of the various genetic markers proposed for premature coronary atherosclerosis is presented in Table 1. These data indicate that the apoA-I/C-III/A-IV gene cluster is a major contributor, particularly because these RFLP sites provide minimal estimates of association due to the variable effects of linkage disequilibrium with a putative etiological locus.

TABLE 1. *Genetic markers for coronary artery disease: relative incidence*

Locus	Relative incidence[a]	Reference
ApoE (E-2/E-3/E-4)	1.17	Cumming & Robertson, 1984 (9)
Lp(a)	2.0	Kostner, 1989 (10)
ApoB (Eco RI site)	2.1	Myant et al., 1989 (11)
LPL (Hind III)	2.92	Chamberlain et al., 1989 (8)
ApoA-I/C-III/A-IV	5.9	Ferns et al., 1985 (4)

[a] Minimal estimates because of linkage disequilibrium.

ACKNOWLEDGMENTS

The author thanks the British Heart Foundation and Medical Research Council (U.K.) for financial support for this project.

REFERENCES

1. Ordovas JM, Cireira F, Pacori M, Jimenez D, Moreda A, Cia P. Apolipoprotein AII, AI, C-III, AIV RFLP frequency and high density lipoprotein cholesterol levels. In: Kostner GM, ed. *Proceedings of the 53rd European Atherosclerosis Society.* Immuno AG: Vienna, 1989:48.
2. Barbir M, Wile D, Trayner I, Thompson GR. High prevalence of hypertriglyceridaemia and apolipoprotein abnormalities in coronary artery disease. *Br Heart J* 1988;60:397–403.
3. Rees A, Stocks J, Sharpe CR, et al. DNA polymorphism in the apolipoprotein AI/CIII gene cluster: association with hypertriglyceridaemia. *J Clin Invest* 1984;76:1090–1095.
4. Ferns GAA, Stocks J, Ritchie C, Galton DJ. Genetic polymorphisms of apolipoprotein CIII and insulin in survivors of myocardial infarction. *Lancet* 1985;1:300–304.
5. Rees A, Jowett NI, Williams LG, et al. DNA polymorphisms flanking the insulin and apolipoprotein CIII genes in atherosclerosis. *Atherosclerosis* 1985;58:269–275.
6. Price WH, Morris SW, Kitchin AH, Wenham PR, Burgon PRS, Donald PM. DNA polymorphisms as markers of familial coronary heart disease. *Lancet* 1989;1:1407–1411.
7. Wim KL, Kirchgessner TG, Lusis AJ, Schotz MC, Lawn RM. Human lipoprotein lipase cDNA sequence. *Science* 1987;235:1638–1641.
8. Chamberlain JC, Thorn JA, Oka K, Galton DJ, Stocks J. DNA polymorphisms at the lipoprotein lipase gene; associations in normal and hypertriglyceridaemic subjects. *Atherosclerosis* 1989;70:85–91.
9. Cumming AM, Robertson SW. Polymorphism at the apo-E locus in relation to risk of coronary artery disease. *Clin Genet* 1984;25:310–313.
10. Kostner GM. Lipoprotein Lp(a) and HMG-CoA reductase inhibitors. *Atherosclerosis* 1989;VIII:405–408.
11. Myant NM, Gallagher J, Thompson GR, Wile D, Humphries SE. RFLP in the apo B gene in relation to coronary heart disease. *Atherosclerosis* 1989;78:9–18.

Atherosclerosis Reviews, Volume 22,
edited by A. M. Gotto, Jr. and R. Paoletti.
Raven Press, Ltd., New York © 1991.

The Insulin Resistance Syndrome

An Epidemiological Overview

P. M. McKeigue

*Department of Community Medicine, University College and Middlesex School of
Medicine, London WC1E 6EA, England*

Metabolic and epidemiologic studies have identified a pattern of associations between plasma triglyceride (TG), insulin, high-density lipoprotein (HDL) cholesterol, glucose intolerance, hypertension, and increased cardiovascular disease (CVD) risk. The lipoprotein disturbances seen in non–insulin-dependent diabetics occur also in individuals with impaired glucose tolerance, in normoglycemic hypertensives, and in otherwise healthy individuals in association with a pattern of obesity in which fat is deposited mainly on the abdomen and trunk. It is now possible to define a syndrome consisting of central obesity, elevated insulin and TG levels, low HDL cholesterol, a tendency to hypertension and glucose intolerance, and increased coronary heart disease (CHD) risk (1).

Although the mechanisms are not fully understood, resistance to insulin-stimulated glucose uptake has a major role in these disturbances. Metabolic studies suggest that the elevated TG levels associated with the insulin resistance syndrome result from a combination of hyperinsulinemia and failure to suppress plasma free fatty acid (FFA) levels, causing increased synthesis of very-low-density lipoprotein (VLDL) TG. Mobilization of central fat stores, by dietary restriction or increased physical activity, alleviates insulin resistance and the metabolic disturbances associated with it. Although the mechanism by which it causes insulin resistance is not understood, central obesity appears to play a primary role in this syndrome.

The insulin resistance syndrome provides a possible unifying explanation for the association of glucose intolerance with disturbances of lipoprotein metabolism and CHD risk. The syndrome may also help to explain high CHD mortality in groups such as South Asians (2) and Scottish men (3). Although central obesity, elevated TG, low HDL cholesterol, hyperinsulinemia, hypertension, and glucose intolerance are all predictors of CHD, with current epidemiological methods it is difficult to distinguish which of these factors are directly related to atherogenesis. The increased CVD risk as-

97

sociated with the insulin resistance syndrome has been explained by the presence of a "cluster of risk factors"; an alternative explanation is that some of these factors predict CHD simply because they are associated with the syndrome. The statistical methods usually employed to test for independent predictors of CHD incidence cannot reliably distinguish the possible causal effects of intercorrelated but labile measurements such as plasma insulin and TG. In multivariate analyses those factors that can be reliably characterized by a single measurement, such as HDL cholesterol, tend to emerge as "independent" predictors more consistently than more labile measurements, such as TG. This does not necessarily mean that low HDL cholesterol is causally related to CHD risk and that elevated TG is not. Comparisons between men and women and between different ethnic groups can help to illuminate some of this confusion and clarify possible causal pathways.

Several of the putative CHD risk factors associated with the insulin resistance syndrome—central body fat, elevated plasma TG, and low plasma HDL cholesterol—display marked sex differences; generally, women have a more favorable distribution than men. Only a few prospective studies of CHD in women are available, but their findings suggest that the insulin resistance syndrome may be especially important in the etiology of CHD in women. In the Framingham Study, glucose intolerance, obesity, elevated TG, and low HDL cholesterol were stronger predictors of CHD incidence in women than in men. The relative immunity of women to CHD is lost in diabetics. In the Gothenburg Studies, central obesity was a more powerful predictor of CHD in women than in men. These findings suggest that metabolic disturbances associated with insulin resistance may be part of the explanation for sex differences in cardiovascular disease risk.

Our studies of the epidemiology of CHD and diabetes in South Asians (Indians, Pakistanis, and Bangladeshis) have led us to emphasize the importance of insulin resistance in this group (2,4). Prevalence of non–insulin-dependent diabetes among urban South Asians settled overseas is ~20% in middle age, compared with 5% in Europeans. CHD mortality in South Asian men and women in the U.K. is 50% higher than in the native British population. This high CHD risk has also been reported for other overseas South Asian populations, and it is unexplained by smoking, plasma cholesterol, or blood pressure (5).

Our preliminary results from a large population survey of men in west London confirm earlier findings of extreme hyperinsulinemia after a glucose load in South Asians compared with Europeans, accompanied by high plasma TG and low HDL cholesterol. These metabolic disturbances are associated with a striking tendency in South Asians to central obesity, as measured by the waist-hip circumference ratio, without any ethnic difference in body mass index. Despite the markedly higher insulin levels after a glucose load in South Asians, FFA levels are not suppressed to the same extent as they are in Europeans. In European men, diminished suppression of FFA levels by a glucose load is associated with central obesity. In both ethnic groups, plasma TG levels are strongly related to the combination of hyper-insulinemia with failure to suppress FFA; this finding is consistent with other studies. These results suggest a possible mechanism for the relationship between body fat pattern and disturbances of lipoprotein metabolism.

The epidemiology of diabetes and CHD in Afro-Caribbeans and African-Americans presents a paradox for the insulin resistance hypothesis, which predicts that high rates of non–insulin-dependent diabetes mellitus will also be accompanied by high CHD risk. Prevalence surveys indicate that diabetes is at least twice as common in Afro-Caribbeans and African-Americans as in whites. However, despite the high prevalence of diabetes and hyperten-sion in blacks, CHD mortality among black men in the U.S.A. and the U.K. is consistently lower than in men of European origin, except in exceptionally deprived inner-city populations where all-cause mortality is high. The ex-planation may lie in the unusually favorable lipoprotein pattern of black men. In American studies, black men have markedly lower plasma TG and higher HDL cholesterol than white men. Our own studies confirm this for Afro-Caribbean men in the U.K. and suggest that insulin resistance does not account for the high diabetes prevalence in this group. A difference in body fat distribution between Afro-Caribbean and European men may also un-derlie the favorable lipoprotein pattern in Afro-Caribbeans.

Other disturbances of lipid metabolism that may be atherogenic and have been described in association with the insulin resistance syndrome include elevated levels of intermediate-density lipoproteins and altered composition of the LDL particle. Rational strategies for preventing the increased CHD risk associated with the insulin resistance syndrome should be based on efforts to reverse the underlying disturbance, rather than treating only the effects on lipids, glucose tolerance, or blood pressure. Increased physical activity and control of obesity offer the best chances of achieving this.

REFERENCES

1. Reaven GM. Role of insulin resistance in human disease. *Diabetes* 1988;37:1595–1607.
2. McKeigue PM, Marmot MG, Syndercombe Court YD, Cottier DE, Rahman S, Riemersma RA. Diabetes, hyperinsulinaemia and coronary risk factors in Bangladeshis in East London. *Br Heart J* 1988;60:390–396.
3. Logan RL, Riemersma RA, Thomson M, et al. Risk factors for ischaemic heart disease in normal men aged 40. Edinburgh-Stockholm Study. *Lancet* 1978;1:949–955.
4. McKeigue PM, Miller GJ, Marmot MG. Coronary heart disease in South Asians overseas—a review. *J Clin Epidemiol* 1989;42:597–609.
5. Beckles GLA, Miller GJ, Kirkwood BR, Alexis SD, Carson DC, Byam NTA. High total and cardiovascular disease mortality in adults of Indian descent in Trinidad, unexplained by major coronary risk factors. *Lancet* 1986;1:1298–1301.

Atherosclerosis Reviews, Volume 22,
edited by A. M. Gotto, Jr. and R. Paoletti.
Raven Press, Ltd., New York © 1991.

Plasma Triglycerides and Cardiovascular Risk in the Population of Mauritius with High Prevalence of Non–Insulin-Dependent Diabetes Mellitus

Jaakko Tuomilehto, *K. George M. M. Alberti,
†Gary Dowse, ‡Farojdeo Hemraj, ‡Djamil Fareed,
‡Hassam Gareeboo, ‡Pierrot Chitson, Zhang Min, and
†Paul Zimmet

*Department of Epidemiology, National Public Health Institute, 00510 Helsinki,
Finland; *University of Newcastle-upon-Tyne, Newcastle-upon-Tyne, England;
†Lions International Diabetes Institute, Caulfield General Medical Centre,
Melbourne, Australia; and ‡Ministry of Health of Mauritius,
Port Louis, Mauritius*

Diabetes is often associated with dyslipidemia. Recent studies have shown that hyperinsulinemia increases plasma triglycerides (TG) and lowers HDL cholesterol (HDL) in subjects both with and without non–insulin-dependent diabetes mellitus (NIDDM) (1–3). The importance of high TG is still poorly understood. Previously, it was thought that there was insufficient evidence to justify treatment of otherwise healthy people with high TG (4). However, this assumption has recently been challenged (5).

Some investigators have suggested that insulin resistance and hyperinsulinemia play central roles in the development of multiple risk factor clusters that lead to coronary heart disease (CHD), but there is little population-based data to confirm this hypothesis (3). We screened a large representative sample of the middle-aged population of Mauritius to determine the levels of noncommunicable disease (NCD) risk factors in Mauritius. We found a very high prevalence of NIDDM (12.1% in men and 11.7% in women aged 25–74 years) among all four ethnic groups (6). In this article, we describe some characteristics of plasma TG levels and CHD risk in Mauritius.

MATERIALS AND METHODS

The target population (aged 25–74 years) and survey methods have been described elsewhere in detail (6). The four major ethnic groups living in

TABLE 1. Age-adjusted mean values of plasma lipids by ethnic group and sex among Mauritians aged 25–64 years

Sex/lipid parameter	Ethnic group			
	Hindu	Muslim	Creole	Chinese
Men				
Total cholesterol	5.6	5.7	5.7	5.3
HDL cholesterol	1.3	1.2	1.3	1.1
Non-HDL cholesterol	4.3	4.5	4.4	4.1
Triglycerides	1.9	1.9	1.7	1.6
Women				
Total cholesterol	5.3	5.3	5.7	5.0
HDL cholesterol	1.3	1.3	1.3	1.4
Non-HDL cholesterol	4.0	4.0	4.4	3.6
Triglycerides	1.2	1.4	1.3	1.0

$p < 0.01$.

Mauritius are Asian Indians–Hindus (54%), Muslims (16%), Creoles (28%), and Chinese (2%). The participation rate approached 90%. Electrocardiograms (ECGs) were recorded and coded for Minnesota code in subjects aged 35 to 74 years. Plasma total cholesterol, TG, HDL cholesterol, and uric acid were determined from fresh specimens in a local laboratory in Mauritius on the same day the samples had been taken. Plasma glucose was also determined fasting and 2 hr after a 75-g load with glucose monohydrate on site with a YSI glucose analyser. Fasting and postload insulin were determined from frozen sera in Newcastle-upon-Tyne where other biochemical determinations were done in a random sample of frozen plasma for quality control purposes. The definitions for "normal" and "abnormal" values for different parameters followed generally adopted criteria. High TG was defined as $\geq$ 2.3 mmol/L and low HDL as $\leq$ 0.9 mmol/L.

TABLE 2. Age-adjusted mean plasma triglycerides by diabetic status among Mauritians aged 25–74 years

Ethnic group	Mean plasma triglycerides (mmol/L)					
	Men			Women		
	Normal	IGT	Diabetic	Normal	IGT	Diabetic
Hindu	1.7	2.3	2.3	1.1	1.4	1.9
Muslim	1.7	2.4	2.5	1.2	1.4	2.2
Creole	1.6	2.1	2.4	1.2	1.4	1.8
Chinese	1.6	2.1	2.4	0.9	1.2	1.5
All	1.6	2.1	2.4	1.1	1.4	1.9

Analysis of covariance: sex, $p < 0.0001$; diabetes status, $p < 0.0001$; interaction: sex–ethnic group–diabetic status, $p = 0.014$.

TABLE 3. *Age-adjusted prevalence of high plasma triglycerides (≥2.3 mmol/L) by ethnic group among Mauritians aged 25–64 years*

Ethnic group	Men		Women	
	%	95% CI	%	95% CI
Hindu	24	21–26	10	8–11
Muslim	25	20–30	8	5–11
Creole	20	16–24	9	7–11
Chinese	12	8–14	8	4–12

CI = confidence interval.

RESULTS

Age-adjusted mean plasma lipids varied little between the ethnic groups: the overall lipid profile was more favorable in Chinese than in the other groups (Table 1). Women had ~40% lower TG levels than men. Glucose intolerance status was a strong determinant of TG (Table 2). TG levels were markedly different between men and women: TG levels in men with impaired glucose tolerance (IGT) were almost as high as among diabetics whereas in women with IGT, TG levels were only slightly elevated as compared with normoglycenic subjects. The prevalence of high TG (> 2.3 mmol/L) was clearly higher in men than in women and it varied only slightly between ethnic groups (Table 3), except the exception of Chinese men who had a markedly lower prevalence.

The prevalence of high TG increased linearly with plasma insulin and was steeper with fasting than it was 2 hr postload insulin (Table 4). At each level of plasma insulin, the male/female prevalence ratio of high TG was about the same. As expected, TG also depended on waist/hip ratio (WHR). The effect of WHR on TG increased with increasing fasting insulin and vice versa (Table 5). Compared with the lowest quartile of both WHR and insulin, the mean TG in the highest quartile of WHR and insulin increased 2.7-fold in men and 2.3-fold in women. In the lowest WHR quartile, TG was the same for both sexes.

Table 6 shows the determinants of high TG in a multivariate model with

TABLE 4. *Prevalence of high triglycerides (≥2.3 mmol/L) by quartiles of serum insulin among Mauritians aged 25–64 years*

Insulin quartile	Fasting		2-Hr postload	
	Men (%)	Women (%)	Men (%)	Women (%)
Q1	8.8	3.2	14.3	8.1
Q2	15.3	5.5	20.2	5.6
Q3	28.5	8.0	26.3	8.9
Q4	43.5	17.5	36.4	12.8

TABLE 5. *Age-adjusted plasma triglycerides (mmol/L) by waist/hip ratio and fasting insulin among Mauritians aged 25–64 years*

	Fasting insulin quartile	Waist/hip ratio		
		Quartile I	Quartile II–III	Quartile IV
Men	I	1.0	1.3	1.6
	II–III	1.1	1.6	2.1
	IV	0.6	2.2	2.7
Women	I	0.9	1.2	1.4
	II–III	1.0	1.3	1.5
	IV	1.3	1.6	2.1

ANOVA: sex, $p = 0.03$; WHR, $p = 0.0001$; insulin, $p = 0.0001$; interaction of sex-WHR-insulin, $p = 0.0001$.

eight other variables. Non-HDL cholesterol, uric acid, and WHR were the strongest independent predictors of high TG. The age-adjusted prevalence of ECG abnormalities suggesting CHD was slightly but not significantly increased in subjects with high TG (Table 7). Analysis of variance showed that TG was particularly high in subjects with diabetes and ECG abnormalities, but the interaction did not reach the level of statistical significance.

COMMENT

Our study showed that the mean level of TG and the prevalence of high TG in Mauritius was higher in men than women. TG was similarly increased in diabetic subjects in both sexes and all four ethnic groups. There is increasing evidence that high TG may be associated with the risk of CHD in diabetic subjects (5,7–9). In Mauritius, the cross-sectional data seem to agree with these previous findings.

The marked effect of hyperinsulinemia on TG levels was further strength-

TABLE 6. *Logistic regression of high triglycerides (TG)[a] on selected parameters among Mauritians aged 25–74 years*

	Men ($n = 2,016$)		Women ($n = 2,302$)	
Parameter	χ^2	p Value	χ^2	p Value
Body mass index	8.8	<0.003	—	n.s.
Waist/hip ratio	22.1	<0.0001	20.1	0.0001
Fasting insulin (log)	8.8	0.003	18.8	<0.0001
2-hr insulin (log)	0.1	n.s.	—	n.s.
Fasting glucose	14.3	0.0002	—	—
Non–HDL cholesterol	52.0	<0.0001	45.0	<0.0001
Uric acid	38.9	<0.0001	21.0	0.0001
Age	19.6	<0.0001	—	n.s.

[a] High TG = plasma TG $\geq$ 2.3 mmol.

TABLE 7. *Age-adjusted prevalence of ischemic ECG abnormalities among Mauritians aged 35–64 years*

	High TG		Normal TG	
	%	95% CI	%	95% CI
Men	19.2	14.7–23.7	15.5	13.4–17.7
Women	39.8	32.1–47.3	32.4	29.9–34.9

CI = confidence interval.

ened by the increase in WHR. Other independently significant determinants of high TG included non-HDL cholesterol and uric acid.

It is commonly agreed that the risk of CHD is due to the clustering of risk factors associated with insulin resistance (10,11). High TG is a relatively good indicator of such a cluster because high TG is the commonest lipid abnormality found in NIDDM, as also shown by our study. This is due to the direct relationship between hyperinsulinemia and high TG through increased hepatic synthesis of very-low-density lipoprotein (1,11).

The controversial question of whether high TG constitutes an independent contributor to the risk of CHD has been clarified by recent prospective data that also included information on older people and HDL in the analyses (5,12). In people over 50 years of age, high TG, when associated with low HDL, has been shown to increase the risk of CHD markedly. Populations with high risk of NIDDM, such as Mauritians, can provide important new information about the role of high TG in the multifactorial and complex etiology of CHD in people with different degrees of glucose intolerance.

REFERENCES

1. Sandek CD, Eder HA. Lipid metabolism in diabetes mellitus. *Am J Med* 1979;66:843–851.
2. Barrett-Connor E, Grundy SM, Holdbrook JJ. Plasma lipids and diabetes mellitus in an adult community. *Am J Epidemiol* 1982;115–163.
3. Zavaroni I, Bonora E, Pagliara M, et al. Risk factors for coronary artery disease in healthy persons with hyperinsulinemia and normal glucose tolerance. *N Engl J Med* 1989;320:702–706.
4. Hulley SB, Rosenman RH, Bawol RD, et al. Epidemiology as a guide to clinical decisions: the association between triglyceride and coronary heart disease. *N Engl J Med* 1980;302:1383–1389.
5. Austin M. Plasma triglyceride as a risk factor for coronary heart disease. The epidemiologic evidence and beyond. *Am J Epidemiol* 1989;129:249–259.
6. Dowse G, Gareeboo H, Zimmet P, et al. High prevalence of NIDDM and impaired glucose tolerance in Indian, Creole and Chinese Mauritians. *Diabetes* 1989;39:390–396.
7. Janka HU. Five-year incidence of major macrovascular complications in diabetes mellitus. *Horm Metabol Res Suppl* 1985;15:15–19.
8. West KM, Ahuja MMS, Bennett PH, et al. The role of circulating glucose and triglyceride concentrations and their interaction with other risk factors as determinants of arterial disease in nine diabetic population samples from the WHO Multinational Study. *Diabetes Care* 1983;6:361–369.
9. Fontbonne A, Eschwège E, Cambien F, et al. Hypertriglyceridaemia as a risk factor of

coronary heart disease mortality in subjects with impaired glucose tolerance or diabetes. *Diabetologia* 1989;32:300–304.

10. Colwell JA, Winocour PD, Lopes-Virella M, Halushka PV. New concepts about the pathogenesis of atherosclerosis in diabetes mellitus. *Am J Med* 1983;75:67–80. –

11. Reaven GM. Role of insulin resistance in human disease. *Diabetes* 1981;30 (suppl 2):66–75. –

12. Abbot RD, Carrol R. Interpreting multiple logistic regression coefficients in prospective observational studies. *Am J Epidemiol* 1983;229:830–836.

Atherosclerosis Reviews, Volume 22,
edited by A. M. Gotto, Jr. and R. Paoletti.
Raven Press, Ltd., New York © 1991.

Dyslipidemic Hypertension in Families with Hypertension, Non–Insulin-Dependent Diabetes Mellitus, and Coronary Heart Disease

R. R. Williams, S. C. Hunt, L. L. Wu, P. N. Hopkins,
M. C. Schumacher, S. Elbein, S. Hasstedt, J. M. Lalouel,
B. M. Stults, and H. Kuida

*Cardiovascular Genetics Research, University of Utah,
Salt Lake City, Utah 84108*

Familial dyslipidemic hypertension (FDH) was first observed among population-based sibships with hypertension in Utah. Basic characteristics of the syndrome include two or more siblings that have both hypertension before the age of 60 years and lipid abnormalities [ninetieth-percentile elevations of cholesterol or triglycerides (TG) and/or tenth-percentile depression of high-density lipoprotein (HDL) cholesterol]. Further characterization of persons with FDH showed that they also have hyperinsulinemia, central obesity, high apoB, low apolipoprotein (apo) A-I and higher frequency of dense low-density lipoprotein (LDL) subfractions. About one-third have familial combined hyperlipidemia (FCHL). In a second study, this syndrome was found among 21% of population-based early coronary families in Utah (ascertained from two or more siblings with coronary disease before the age of 55 years).

In a third study of 173 family members with normal glucose tolerance in 14 large Utah pedigrees with two or more siblings with non–insulin-dependent diabetes mellitus (NIDDM), dyslipidemia was common, 25% were hypertensive, and dyslipidemic hypertension (DH) was found in 18%. Compared to normotensive controls, 1-hr–stimulated insulin levels were higher among both obese and nonobese persons with DH in NIDDM families.

In summary, FDH appears to be a subtype of essential hypertension due to metabolic abnormalities that are precursors of hypertension, NIDDM, and early familial coronary heart disease (CHD). Population-based data from Utah suggest FDH occurs in 2% of the general population, 12% of hypertensive subjects, 21% of patients with early familial CHD, and 18% of normoglycemic relatives of NIDDM. Additional research is needed to determine the primary pathophysiologic mechanisms of FDH, including the degree to which these manifestations can be attributed to specific segregating major genes, blended polygenes, shared family environment, or combinations of these predetermining factors.

MATERIALS AND METHODS

A "Health Family Tree" questionnaire collected from the parents of Utah high school students between 1983 and 1986 identified 222,546 living adults (1). Of these living adults, 3% reported having medicated high blood pressure (HBP) and another sibling with HBP, both diagnosed before the age of 60 years. Of these available hypertensive siblings, 131 participants from 58 sibships attended the Cardiovascular Genetics Research Clinic at the University of Utah for detailed evaluation (2).

From the same questionnaires, we identified 474 persons with coronary disease before age 55 in sibships with two or more affected brothers or sisters; 44 of them have attended the Cardiovascular Genetics Research Clinic (3).

The observed frequency of lipid abnormalities was compared to the norm for the Lipid Research Clinics (LRC) population using a χ^2 analysis for statistical significance. For total cholesterol, LDL cholesterol, and TG, abnormal levels were defined as those above the ninetieth or ninety-fifth percentile of the Lipid Research Clinics data (4). For HDL cholesterol, values below the 10th or 5th percentile of the LRC data were considered abnormal. The Utah lipid laboratory has been standardized to an LRC laboratory (5).

TABLE 1. *Frequency of dyslipidemia and obesity in 131 siblings with early familial hypertension*

Abnormality	Observed frequency		Ratio of observed to expected	
	90th[a]	95th[b]	90th[a]	95th[b]
1. Low HDL cholesterol	39%	21%	3.9[c]	4.2[c]
2. High triglycerides	30%	18%	3.0[c]	3.6[c]
3. High LDL cholesterol	19%	13%	1.9[d]	2.6[c]
Any of the above lipid abnormalities	65%	47%	2.4[c]	3.4[c]
4. High ideal weight[e]	29%	13%	2.9[c]	2.6[c]

[a] Columns contain results with "abnormal" defined as HDL ≤ 10th percentile and LDL cholesterol or TG ≥ 90th percentile compared to the Lipid Research Clinics data ($n = 48,482$).

[b] Columns contain results using HDL ≤ 5th percentile and LDL cholesterol or TG ≥ 95th percentile as abnormal.

[c] $p < 0.00001$ (from χ^2 statistic).

[d] $p < 0.001$ (from χ^2 statistic).

[e] Percentiles of ideal weight were based on normotensive controls ($n = 391$).

TABLE 2. *Subsets of familial dysplipidemic hypertension (FDH) patients compared to normolipidemic hypertensives for metabolic variables*

Variables	Values in normolipidemic hypertensives	Ratio of mean in FDH vs. normolipidemic hypertensives		
		FDH with FCHL		Other FDH
Males/females	10/10	8/11		22/22
LDL-cholesterol	136 mg/dl	1.22^a	<>	1.04
VLDL-cholesterol	13 mg/dl	2.96^c		2.22^c
HDL-cholesterol	50 mg/dl	0.83^b	<>	0.67^c
ApoB	91 mg/dl	1.33^c	<>	1.19^b
ApoA-I	98 mg/dl	1.05	<>	0.92
LDL subfraction	2.93 band 1–7	1.36^b		1.36^b
Fasting insulin	12.0 mU/l	1.73^b		1.48^a
Fasting glucose	90.2 mg/dl	1.18		1.14
Body mass index	27.4 kg/m^2	1.04	<>	1.15^b
Scap skinfold	23.2 mm	1.19		1.28^a
Knee width	91.8 mm	1.01	<>	1.08^a
Wrist circumference	15.0 mm	1.03	<>	1.17^c

<> denotes significant difference ($p < 0.05$) beteen FDH subsets (FCHL vs. other).
[a] $p < 0.05$, [b] $p < 0.01$, [c] $p < 0.001$, for each FDH subset vs. normolipidemic HBP.

RESULTS

Table 1 shows excess dyslipidemia and obesity in the hypertensive siblings (2). Familial aggregation of dyslipidemia in HBP sibships was also significantly higher than expected ($p < 0.00001$). Based on the data recorded in Table 1, a new syndrome termed "familial dyslipidemic hypertension" (FDH) was defined as a family where two or more siblings were diagnosed before age 60 with hypertension accompanied by abnormalities in either TG, cholesterol, or HDL cholesterol (2). As shown in Table 2, significantly in-

TABLE 3. *Frequency of dyslipidemic or 20 coronary heart disease (CHD) sibships with 44 siblings having CHD before age 55*

Dyslipidemia syndrome	Frequency of syndrome	
	CHD sibships	General population
1. Familial combined hyperlipidemia		
LDL cholesterol and TG ≥ 90th percentile	30%	1–2%
Total cholesterol and TG ≥ 90th percentile	40%	2–3%
2. Familial dyslipidemic hypertension		
2 Sibs dyslipidemic and 2 HBP	15%	1–2%
2 Sibs dyslipidemic and 1 HBP	45%	3–4%
3. Low HDL cholesterol (normal total cholesterol)	10%	0.5–1%
(HDL cholesterol ≤ 10th, total cholesterol ≥ 90th)		
4. Type III hyperlipidemia	5%	0.2–0.5%
ApoE 2/2; VLDL cholesterol/TG > 0.30)		
5. Early CHD with normal lipids	15%	0.5–1%

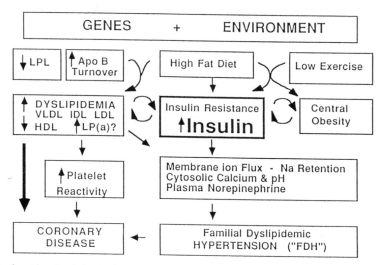

FIG. 1. A pathophysiological model suggesting the possible mechanisms and interrelationships by which both genetic and environmental factors could help promote the metabolic abnormalities common to dyslipidemic hypertension, early coronary disease, and insulin resistance.

creased very-low-density lipoprotein (VLDL) cholesterol and fasting plasma insulin levels were observed in two subsets of patients with FDH (6). Those who met criteria for FCHL had prominent elevations in apoB, whereas the members of the other subgroup had central obesity, low HDL cholesterol, low apoA-I levels, and above-average measurements of the bony structures (6).

The frequency of FDH and other lipid syndromes in sibships with two or more cases of early CHD is presented in Table 3 (3). In 15% of early CHD sibships, two dyslipidemic hypertensive subjects were found, whereas 45% of sibships had two dyslipidemic persons of whom at least one had HBP (3). Sibships with FDH often had FCHL or low HDL cholesterol.

DISCUSSION

A possible pathophysiological model relating all these abnormalities to each other is presented in Fig. 1. There are at least four mechanisms that could explain how hyperinsulinemia promotes HBP: renal sodium retention, increased norepinephrine, hypertrophy of vascular smooth muscle, and increased cytosolic free calcium (7). Many individuals show only the abnormalities in lipids or insulin, whereas some also have HBP, diabetes, and CHD. Fourteen Utah pedigrees ascertained for two individuals with type II diabetes show abnormalities in lipids and insulin in many first-degree relatives with normal glucose tolerance tests. Hypertension is also found more often than expected in these relatives of families with type II diabetes (unpublished Utah data, 1990). Dyslipidemic HBP was seen in 18% of them, and 72% of all hypertensive relatives of NIDDM had dyslipidemic HBP.

In persons with FDH, risk of early familial CHD may derive largely from the metabolic abnormality rather than the elevated blood pressure. This might help explain why HBP treatment trials only show about one-half of the benefit expected from prospective studies (8). It seems prudent for physicians treating persons with hypertension to look for lipid abnormalities by measuring cholesterol, TG, and HDL cholesterol. To prevent early coronary disease most effectively, the lipid abnormality should be treated and followed at least as carefully as hypertension.

REFERENCES

1. Williams RR, Hunt SC, Barlow GK, et al. Health family trees: a tool for finding and helping young family members of coronary and cancer prone pedigrees in Texas and Utah. *Am J Public Health* 1988;78:1283–1286.
2. Williams RR, Hunt SC, Hopkins PN, et al. Familial dyslipidemic hypertension: evidence from 58 Utah families for a syndrome present in approximately 12% of patients with essential hypertension. *JAMA* 1988;259:3579–3586.
3. Williams RR, Hopkins PN, Hunt SC, et al. Population-based frequency of dyslipidemia syndromes in coronary prone families in Utah. *Arch Intern Med* 1990;150:582–588.
4. The Prevalence Study, vol 1. In: *Lipid Research Clinics population studies data book*. National Institutes of Health publication 80-1527. Washington, D.C.: U.S. Dept. of Health and Human Services, Public Health Service, 1980.
5. Wu LL, Warnick GR, Wu JT, Williams RR, Lalouel JM. A rapid micro-scale procedure for determination of the total lipid profile. *Clin Chem* 1989;35:1486–1491.
6. Hunt SC, Wu LL, Hopkins PN, et al. Apolipoprotein, low density lipoprotein subfraction, and insulin associations with familial combined hyperlipidemia: study of Utah patients with familial dyslipidemic hypertension. *Arteriosclerosis* 1989;9:335–344.
7. Kaplan NM. The deadly quartet: upper-body obesity, glucose intolerance, hypertriglyceridemia, and hypertension. *Arch Intern Med* 1989;149:1514–1520.
8. Collins R, Peto R, MacMahon S, et al. Blood pressure, stroke, and coronary artery disease. *Lancet* 1990;335:765–774,827–838.

Atherosclerosis Reviews, Volume 22,
edited by A. M. Gotto, Jr. and R. Paoletti.
Raven Press, Ltd., New York © 1991.

Abdominal Obesity and Risk for Cardiovascular Disease and Diabetes

P. Björntorp

Department of Medicine I and the Wallenberg Laboratory, Sahlgren's Hospital, University of Göteborg, Sweden

Recent epidemiological research has demonstrated the strong predictive power of the waist/hip circumference ratio (WHR) for the development of cardiovascular disease (CVD) and non–insulin-dependent diabetes mellitus (NIDDM). This new risk factor shows the same independent strength in prediction for the aforementioned diseases as previously established risk factors such as cholesterol, high blood pressure, smoking, and insulin dependence, and it applies to both sexes. The WHR is an anthropometric measurement that describes the distribution of body fat mainly to central (high WHR) or peripheral (low WHR) adipose tissue regions.

With an elevated WHR, the risk for CVD and NIDDM seems to be independent of obesity, but WHR is synergistic with obesity for risk to NIDDM. In contrast, epidemiological studies show that the risk for CVD with WHR is actually inversely dependent on obesity; in other words, otherwise lean subjects with a high WHR would have the highest risk to develop CVD. These opposite influences of obesity and WHR on the likelihood of developing CVD might provide an explanation for the controversial results obtained by investigators who have analyzed CVD risk in relation to obesity alone. It should also be noted that even though WHR is an independent predictor of CVD, it is also strongly statistically correlated to the other established risk factors for CVD (i.e., blood lipids, high blood pressure, smoking, insulin, fibrinogen, etc.). [For a more detailed review of this research, see ref. 1.]

EPIDEMIOLOGICAL STUDIES

Very recent analyses of the relationship of WHR to CVD for both men and women in ongoing epidemiological studies in Göteborg, Sweden, have focused on the association of this risk factor with sex differences in cases of myocardial infarction (MI). Some differences between male and female subjects were found for such established strong risk factors as cholesterol, blood pressure, and smoking. The risk for CVD (odds ratio) was about three times higher in men than women. When the differences in cholesterol, blood pressure, and smoking were adjusted for, the odds ratio remained essentially the same. When, however, the WHR was introduced into the adjustments, whether in combination with the other risk factors, or alone, the odds ratio was close to unity; in other words, the sex-related risk to develop CVD had disappeared. Other analyses showed correlations between WHR and selective risk for CVD with the same regression coefficient. The regression lines overlapped where the WHR distribution for women and men also overlapped. This analysis thus demonstrates again the significance of the WHR as a risk factor for CVD development. It suggests that the sex differences seen at middle age may actually be explained by the WHR or at least by a factor closely related to this ratio (2).

PATHOGENETIC MECHANISMS

The statistical relationship between the WHR and the endpoints CVD and NIDDM could be either coincidental, parallel, or causative. Given the consistency of these findings, it seems highly unlikely that it is coincidental. It may, however, be a parallel or causative phenomenon. The WHR is a complex measurement made up of such components as pelvis width, local muscle mass, intestinal contents, as well as subcutaneous and intraabdominal fat. Although prospective analyses of the relative risk of these individual components are not available, several recent studies performed independently in different laboratories and focusing on these particular adipose tissues in relation to CVD and NIDDM risk have shown that the previously established risk factors are most closely associated statistically to the visceral fat mass, as measured with computerized tomography scans (3).

The visceral adipose tissues have a high lipolytic sensitivity; in other words, they release their free fatty acids (FFA) very efficiently. This function seems to be particularly efficient in the tissues drained by the portal vein (omental and mesenteric adipose tissues), especially in normal or obese men and in abdominally obese women. In addition, insulin inhibition of lipolysis is blunted in these tissues. With enlargement of the visceral fat and concomitant increase in fat cells, these factors would combine synergistically to pour FFA into the portal vein in high concentrations. This metabolic alteration may well have a number of untoward consequences.

EFFECT OF PORTAL FFA ON HEPATIC REGULATION
OF METABOLISM

The ability of FFA to increase the synthesis of very-low-density lipoproteins (VLDL) in the liver has long been established. Recent studies have shown that it is actually the delivery of FFA, which form triglycerides (TG) for VLDL transport, rather than the other lipid components or the protein backbone, apolipoprotein B_{100} (apoB$_{100}$) that is rate limiting for the VLDL transport and secretion. This seems to be due to the long half-life of the mRNA for apoB$_{100}$, which allows an excess of apoB$_{100}$ translation. It follows, then, that portal FFA drive the hepatic excretion of VLDL. Under appropriate conditions, this lipoprotein, as well as low-density lipoproteins (LDL) and apoB$_{100}$ will tend to increase in concentration in the circulation.

Fatty acids also stimulate liver gluconeogenesis. Evidence for this is provided in studies of the cellular mechanisms at the enzymatic level, where the activity of pyruvate carboxylase and the reduced state of nucleotides in the β-oxidation of fatty acids have been found to be of particular importance. Studies *in vivo* have demonstrated that the concentration of circulating FFA and their hepatic oxidation are important regulators of hepatic gluconeogenesis. This fact has also, as far as technically and ethically possible, been demonstrated in humans.

An additional important effect of fatty acids on isolated hepatocytes is the inhibition of insulin binding, degradation, and function. Inhibition apparently results from internalization of the insulin receptor in a first step; it is also—like gluconeogenesis—seemingly dependent on fatty acid oxidation. Corresponding findings have been made in the *in situ* perfused intact liver and in overfed rats. Humans with increased visceral fat masses also apparently extract comparably little insulin over the liver. The end result will be that insulin, produced in the pancreatic β-cells and delivered into the portal vein, is transferred to a large extent into the peripheral circulation, creating hyperinsulinemia.

The interrelated mechanisms of oxidation of portal FFA in the liver and hepatic gluconeogenesis may well include a physiological regulatory function that triggers glucose production for the periphery, particularly the brain, during the transition from the absorptive to the postalimentary phases. This function would also be assisted by the shunting of insulin during this process. Delivery of excess lipid energy from the liver to the periphery via VLDL is also an apparently useful physiological regulatory mechanism under normal conditions.

One attractive hypothesis is that these mechanisms, when driven to excess activity by elevated portal FFA concentrations, result in excessive concentrations of glucose, insulin, and VLDL in the systemic circulation. Furthermore, LDL and apoB$_{100}$ would then also tend to be circulating in elevated concentrations, particularly in cases where removal mechanisms are impaired.

Ongoing discussion on the association between hyperinsulinemia, insulin resistance, and hypertension, based on considerable evidence from both epidemiological and experimental studies, suggests that hyperinsulinemia actually causes blood pressure elevation [for reviews see refs. 4 and 5].

Taken together with the tendency of portal FFA to create hyperinsulinemia, hypertension may thus also be linked to the rest of this syndrome.

In summary, fatty acids have been shown to drive VLDL synthesis and gluconeogenesis, as well as to diminish hepatic uptake of insulin. When these mechanisms are exaggerated by high portal FFA concentrations, there may be a risk for increased concentrations of glucose and insulin, as well as VLDL and its derivatives, LDL and apoB$_{100}$. Given the potential association between hyperinsulinemia and hypertension, this mechanism might cause hyperglycemia; hyperinsulinemia; hypertension; and increased concentrations of VLDL, LDL, and apoB$_{100}$. All of these are established risk factors for CVD and NIDDM. The increased lipolytic sensitivity and enlargement of visceral adipose tissues—particularly those drained by the portal vein—might then provide increased portal concentrations of FFA and serve to generate most of the established CVD and NIDDM risk factors. This hypothesis offers a pathogenetic link between visceral fat enlargement, risk factors, and the appropriate disease endpoints. It has recently been reviewed with detailed references (6).

ENDOCRINE ABERRATIONS ASSOCIATED WITH AN INCREASED WHR

Evidence suggests that endocrine aberrations follow the WHR syndrome. The relationship holds for both adrenal corticosteroids and sex steroid hormones in both sexes. Women with WHR have frequent irregular ovulations and menses, with concomitant deficiency of progesterone production. They also may have hyperandrogenicity. In contrast, men have lowered testosterone. There have also been reports of increased cortisol secretion following an abdominal distribution of body fat; this condition is followed by a relative insulin resistance. Of particular interest in this regard is a study that found marked insulin resistance after administration of low doses of testosterone to female rats (7). A low sex hormone–binding globulin concentration, indicating a hyperandrogenic state in women, is a strong risk factor for the development of NIDDM and is closely parallel to fasting insulin concentrations, indicating insulin resistance (8).

Taken together, the aberrations of steroid hormone secretion seen in subjects with abdominal obesity may well by themselves cause the marked insulin resistance seen in this syndrome. There is also evidence that such endocrine aberrations are causative in abdominal fat accumulation (e.g., Cushing's syndrome). The other metabolic derangements might be a consequence of primary insulin resistance, whether or not in combination with the factors discussed in connection with the visceral fat hypothesis. The most likely alternative may actually be a combination of these two mechanisms (9).

REFERENCES

1. Björntorp P. The association between obesity, adipose tissue distribution and disease. *Acta Med Scand* 1988;723(suppl):121–134.
2. Larsson B, Bengtsson C, Björntorp P, et al. Is abdominal body fat distribution a main explanation for the sex difference in the incidence of myocardial infarction? (submitted for publication).
3. Björntorp P. Abdominal obesity and the development of non–insulin dependent diabetes mellitus. *Diabetes Meta Rev* 1988;7:615–622.
4. Björntorp P. Hypertension in obesity. *Acta Med Scand* 1982;211:271–272.
5. Reaven GR, Hoffman BB. A role for insulin in the aetiology and course of hypertension? *Lancet* 1987;2:435–436.
6. Björntorp P. "Portal" adipose tissue as a generator of risk factors in cardiovascular disease and diabetes. *Atherosclerosis* 1990;10:493–496.
7. Holmäng A, Svedberg J, Jennische E, Björntorp P. The effects of testosterone on muscle insulin sensitivity and morphology in female rats. *Am J Physiol* 1990;259:E555–E560.
8. Lindstedt G, Lindberg PA, Lapidus L, Lundgren H, Bengtsson C, Björntorp P. Low sex hormone binding globulin is an independent risk factor for the development of non–insulin dependent diabetes mellitus. A 12-year follow-up of the population study of women in Göteborg, Sweden. *Diabetes* 1991;40:123–128.
9. Björntorp P. Obesity and diabetes. In: Alberti KGMM, Krall LP, eds. *The Diabetes annual*; vol 5, 1991 (in press).

Atherosclerosis Reviews, Volume 22,
edited by A. M. Gotto, Jr. and R. Paoletti.
Raven Press, Ltd., New York © 1991.

Insulin, Glucose Tolerance, Triglycerides, and Coronary Heart Disease

A 12-Year Follow-Up in Normal Men

R. L. Logan, A. Hargreaves, R. A. Riemersma, *R. Elton, K. D. Buchanan, and M. F. Oliver

*Cardiovascular Research Unit and *Department of Medicine, University of Edinburgh, Edinburgh EH8 9XF, Scotland*

The coronary heart disease (CHD) incidence and mortality rates for middle-aged men in Edinburgh in the 1970s were three times those in Stockholm. The Edinburgh-Stockholm Study (1) provided a basis for assessing the relative importance of various risk factors, including the response of insulin to an oral glucose load, to explain this dramatic difference. The study was originally conducted in healthy men within 6 months of their 40th birthday in Edinburgh and Stockholm. The clinical and laboratory measurements were conducted at the same time, and all the laboratory analyses were made in the same laboratories; thus, there were no methodological errors between the laboratories.

In summary, the results showed that the Edinburgh men had a significantly higher elevation of serum triglyceride (TG), very-low-density lipoprotein (VLDL) TG, and low-density lipoprotein (LDL) TG than the Stockholm men. Although the two groups showed no significant difference in total serum cholesterol or LDL cholesterol, high-density-lipoprotein (HDL) cholesterol was significantly lower in Edinburgh men. There was no difference in the glucose response to a standard oral glucose tolerance test ($30g/m^2$). However, Edinburgh men exhibited a greater insulin response (total area under the insulin curve).

Among numerous other differences between the populations, the Edinburgh men were shorter and had a greater body mass (weight/height ratio) and thicker triceps skin folds. The Edinburgh men also had a higher systolic and diastolic blood pressure.

THE 12-YEAR FOLLOW-UP

The Edinburgh-Stockholm Study provided us with an opportunity to conduct a small longitudinal study in Edinburgh men. Of the 107 men in the

TABLE 1. *Baseline measurements of oral glucose tolerance test in 107 Edinburgh men aged 40 years: relationship to subsequent CHD (12-year follow-up) (mean ± SD)*

	No CHD (n = 96)	CHD (n = 11)
Fasting insulin (μU/ml)	6.2 ± 3.4	6.8 ± 3.9
Insulin max (μU/ml)	62 ± 51	72 ± 33
Time to insulin max (min)	52 ± 27	52 ± 31
Insulin area[a] (up to 60 min)	2,371 ± 1,780	2,201 ± 1,150
Insulin area[a] (up to 120 min)	4,395 ± 3,542	4,165 ± 1,641
Fasting glucose (mM)	5.12 ± 0.52	4.95 ± 0.32
Glucose area (up to 60 min)	445 ± 59	426 ± 48
Glucose area (up to 120 min)	822 ± 128	793 ± 101

[a] μU × min/ml.

Edinburgh component of the Edinburgh-Stockholm Study, all were traced for a 12-year follow-up. Of these, 83 underwent a formal interview, a clinical examination, and the same biochemical tests originally made 12 years earlier. Of the cohort of 107, 11 developed CHD. This approximates the expected incidence. No similar follow-up has been conducted in the Swedish men.

Carbohydrate and Insulin in Relation to Subsequent CHD

No relationship was found between subsequent CHD and fasting insulin at baseline, the time to reach maximum insulin secretion, or the maximum insulin level. Similarly, there was no significant relationship between development of CHD and the area under the insulin curve (up to either 60 or 120 min) during the glucose tolerance test (Table 1).

In addition, we found no significant relationship between subsequent CHD and either fasting glucose or glucose area under the glucose curve in response to an oral glucose tolerance test when assessed at baseline (Table 2).

TABLE 2. *Baseline measurements of plasma lipids and selected risk factors in 107 Edinburgh men aged 40 years: relationships to subsequent CHD (12-year follow-up) (mean ± SD)*

Fasting values	No CHD (n = 96)	CHD (n = 11)
Triglycerides (mmol/L)	1.80 ± 1.06	2.07 ± 1.03
Total cholesterol (mmol/L)	5.49 ± 0.91	5.89 ± 0.73
HDL-cholesterol (mmol/L)	1.26 ± 0.26	1.11 ± 0.16[a]
Cholesterol/HDL cholesterol ratio	4.52 ± 1.21	5.45 ± 1.29[a]
Smoking habit (%)	53	91[a]
Weight/height ratio (kg/m²) × 10⁻²	.249 ± 0.003	.267 ± 0.008[a]
Abdominal skinfold (mm)	12.3 ± 0.4	15.8 ± 1.2[a]

[a] $p < 0.05$.

Plasma Lipids and Lipoproteins and Subsequent CHD

Fasting TG and VLDL did not change over the 12 years. There was no relationship between later CHD and fasting TG or TG/HDL ratio at baseline (Table 2), even though a trend was seen in terms of higher TG levels in the CHD patients.

No significant relationship was found between total plasma cholesterol at baseline and the subsequent development of CHD (Table 2). However, there was a borderline significant correlation between LDL and subsequent CHD ($p = 0.053$) and a significant relationship between HDL cholesterol at baseline and later CHD ($p = 0.046$). The total cholesterol/HDL ratio also correlated with subsequent CHD ($p = 0.02$).

Obesity and Subsequent CHD

There was a significant correlation between body mass index and subsequent CHD ($p < 0.05$) (Table 2). We made measurements of central obesity at baseline and found a significant correlation between abdominal skin folds and development of CHD ($p < 0.05$).

Other Risk Factors

The importance of hypertriglyceridemia, insulin, and glucose tolerance cannot be fully assessed without taking other classical risk factors into consideration. The most striking of all relationships between baseline measurements of classical risk factors and subsequent CHD was cigarette smoking; 91% of the patients who eventually developed CHD were smokers, as compared with 53% of those who did not develop CHD.

Multivariate Analysis

Multiple logistic regression was undertaken to examine pairs of factors in combination, incorporating interaction, in order to see whether any two together were more predictive of CHD than could be expected from the additive effects. Although cases of heart disease tended to be associated with low HDL, CHD was not especially frequent in subjects with both low HDL and high insulin. This finding represents a nonsignificant interaction. Similar analyses were done combining different insulin measurements and other lipid fractions, but these calculations also failed to show significant interaction.

DISCUSSION

It is important to emphasize that this small study might not have the statistical significance to predict CHD 12 years after baseline measurements. Although some factors have been shown to be significant predictors of subsequent heart disease, the results are based on a small sample of men who experienced few coronary events. The statistical power of the study is therefore low, and estimation of the actual magnitude of the risk associated with these factors must be imprecise.

For example, the estimated odds ratio for heart disease in those who smoked in 1976 as compared to those who did not is 8.82, but the 95% confidence limits are 1.16 and 384. Similar wide limits also apply to the cases where factors do not show a significant association with heart disease. For example, 6 of 55 men with a TG level of > 1.5 had subsequent heart disease as compared to 5 of 52 with TG < 1.5, giving an odds ratio of 1.15 with 95% confidence limits of 0.27 and 5.11. Thus, although our study is consistent with the hypothesis that high TG confers no excess risk, we cannot rule out the possibility that the odds ratio could be as great as fivefold. Nevertheless, the plasma total HDL cholesterol ratio and cigarette smoking both had predictive value. Therefore, even in a study with small numbers, the influence of cholesterol metabolism and cigarette smoking was significant. The insulin parameters appeared not to be significantly related to CHD, but the confidence limits of the odds ratio were very wide (Table 3).

Some investigators have argued that insulin resistance is a particularly important predictor of CHD. The syndrome that indicates insulin resistance includes raised insulin levels in response to a glucose load, raised TG levels, low HDL cholesterol concentrations, raised systolic blood pressure, and central obesity (2). In larger studies (3–5), raised insulin concentrations have been shown, to be predictive of CHD. But as far as this small study is concerned, none of the various responses of insulin to a glucose load nor their associations with lipoprotein levels correlated significantly with CHD.

TABLE 3. *Estimated odds ratios and 95% confidence intervals (CI) for subsequent CHD from risk factors*

Factor	Odds ratio	95% CI
HDL cholesterol <1.25 mmol/L	4.30	0.82, 42.55
Insulin (60 min area) >1800[a]	0.80	0.15, 4.03
Insulin (120 min area) >3300[a]	3.78	0.65, 39.06
Fasting glucose >5 mmol/L	0.50	0.10, 2.15
Wt/ht index >0.25 kg/m² × 10⁻²	5.32	1.01, 52.36
Systolic BP >135 mm Hg	0.53	0.11, 2.24
Diastolic BP >85 mm Hg	3.65	0.70, 36.10

Cut-off points for risk factors were taken at approximate median.
[a] μU × min/ml.

HDL cholesterol and cigarette smoking appear to be more powerful predictors than measurements of insulin-TG metabolism.

ACKNOWLEDGMENTS

This study was supported by a grant from the Scottish Committee of the Chest, Heart, and Stroke Association. The Cardiovascular Research Unit is supported by the British Heart Foundation.

REFERENCES

1. Logan RL, Riemersma RA, Thomson M, et al. Risk factors for ischaemic heart disease in normal men aged 40. *Lancet* 1978;1:949–955.
2. Reaven GM. Banting Lecture 1988. Role of insulin resistance in human disease. *Diabetes* 1988;37:1595–1607.
3. Ducimetiere P, Eschwege E, Papoz L, et al. Relationship of plasma insulin levels to the incidence of myocardial infarction and coronary heart disease mortality in a middle-aged population. *Diabetologia* 1980;19:205–210.
4. Pyorala K, Savolanainen E, Kaukola S, Haapakoski G. Plasma insulin as coronary heart disease risk factor: relationship to other risk factors and predictive value during $9\frac{1}{2}$ year follow-up of the Helsinki Policemen Study Population. *Acta Med Scand* 1985;701(suppl):38–52.
5. Welborn TA, Wearne K. Coronary heart disease incidence and cardiovascular mortality in Busselton with reference to glucose and insulin concentrations. *Diabetes Care* 1979;2:154–160.

Atherosclerosis Reviews, Volume 22,
edited by A. M. Gotto, Jr. and R. Paoletti.
Raven Press, Ltd., New York © 1991.

Hyperlipidemias and the Fibrinolytic System

L. Mussoni, L. Mannucci, M. Camera, L. Sironi, and E. Tremoli

*Institute of Pharmacological Sciences and E. Grossi Paoletti Center,
University of Milan, Milan, Italy*

The fibrinolytic system dissolves fibrin deposits within the vascular bed. The enzyme responsible for fibrin dissolution is plasmin, which is generated during the *in vivo* activation of the circulating proenzyme plasminogen (1,2). The system is tightly regulated by the availability of activators, i.e., tissue plasminogen activator (t-PA), and inhibitors, such as plasminogen activator inhibitor (PAI-1) (Fig. 1). t-PA and PAI-1 normally circulate in plasma at nanomolar concentrations, these levels being affected, however, in a variety of pathophysiological conditions. In particular, thrombin, insulin, bacterial lipopolysaccharides and growth factors, as well as chemicals such as tumor promoters and retinoids, are among agents known to induce t-PA and PAI-1 synthesis and/or release. Under physiological conditions t-PA generates plasmin preferentially on fibrin surfaces. Recently it has been shown that t-PA and plasminogen specifically bind to receptors present on endothelial cells with the consequent generation of plasmin on the endothelial cell surface (3).

LIPIDS AND FIBRINOLYSIS

The influence of plasma lipids on the fibrinolytic system was first suggested in 1955 by Grieg (4), who demonstrated that fibrinolytic activity was inhibited following a fatty meal—an observation confirmed by some but not all subsequent studies. To understand whether changes in the plasma lipid levels could affect this important defense mechanism against vascular occlusion, a number of studies were performed. In fact, as previously mentioned, the fibrinolytic system is primarily responsible for the dissolution of fibrin deposits into the vascular bed, and its alterations are considered risk factors for thrombotic episodes. The results of studies conducted in normal subjects and patients with different pathological conditions, such as coronary heart disease (CHD), deep venous thrombosis, diabetes, etc. (5–7), suggest

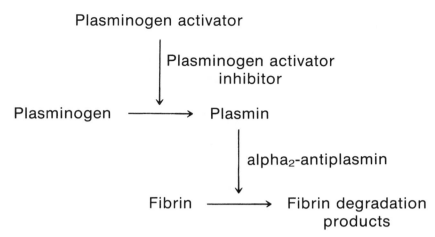

FIG. 1. Schematic representation of the fibrinolytic system.

that triglyceride (TG) levels influence the fibrinolytic system by reducing total fibrinolytic capacity. These findings have been further supported by the results of studies in patients diagnosed with hyperlipidemia who had no history of thromboembolic episodes. In particular, an alteration of the fibrinolytic system has been reported in patients with hypertriglyceridemia, type IV hyperlipoproteinemia according to the Fredrickson classification (8), but not in patients with type IIa or type IIb hypercholesterolemia (Table 1).

As shown in Table 1, in the five studies conducted in patients with type IV hypertriglyceridemia, total fibrinolytic capacity was reduced (9–13). Also, fibrinolytic activity in response to DDAVP was highly impaired in patients with a tendency to develop hyperchilomicronemia (type IV/V) (12). Cucuíanu et al. (10) also studied patients with type IIa and type IIb hyper-

TABLE 1. *Fibrinolysis and hyperlipoproteinemia*

Patient	Number	Stimulus	Assay	Fibrinolytic capacity	References
Type IV	8	Treadmill exercise	ELA	Reduced	Epstein et al., 1970 (9)
Type IV	54	Ergometric bicycle	DBLCT	Reduced	Cuculanu et al., 1979 (10)
Type IIa	30	Ergometric bicycle	DBCLT	Normal	Cuculanu et al., 1979 (10)
Type IIb	51	Ergometric bicycle	DBCLT	Reduced	Cuculanu et al., 1979 (10)
Type IV	20	Venous occlusion	ELT	Reduced	Andersen et al., 1981 (11)
Type IIa	17	Venous occlusion	ELT	Normal	Andersen et al., 1981 (11)
Type IIb	47	Venous occlusion	ELT	Normal	Andersen et al., 1981 (11)
Type IV/V	10	DDAVP	ELA	Reduced	Brommer et al., 1982 (12)
Type IIb/IV	8	DDAVP	ELA	Normal	Brommer et al., 1982 (12)
Type IV	18	DDAVP	DBCLT	Reduced	Simpson et al., 1983 (13)

ELA: euglobulin lysis area; ELT: euglobulin lysis time; DDAVP: 1-desamino-8-D-arginine vasopressin (desmopressin); DBCLT: dilluted blood clot lysis time.

lipoproteinemia. Fibrinolytic capacity was found to be reduced in patients with type IIb but not type IIa hyperlipoproteinemia. In contrast, Andersen et al. (11) found total fibrinolytic activity within normal levels also in type IIb patients.

In some of these studies an inverse correlation was found between TG levels and fibrinolytic capacity. On the other hand, a direct correlation between TG and plasma levels of PAI-1, the major circulating inhibitor of t-PA, was noted in survivors of myocardial infarction (MI) (5,14).

In recent years, it has emerged that the components of the fibrinolytic system may be affected by a number of factors, such as diurnal variations, age, body mass index, insulin levels, etc. On the other hand, patients with hypertriglyceridemia may easily have alterations in carbohydrate metabolism as well as increased body weight. In addition, to the best of our knowledge, the single components of this system have not been determined in any of the studies carried out in patients with hypertriglyceridemia and no thromboembolic complications.

In a study recently carried out in our Lipid Clinic (15), total fibrinolytic activity as well as t-PA and PAI-1 antigen and activities were evaluated in a group of patients with type IV hyperlipoproteinemia. The results were compared to those obtained in a group of normolipidemic subjects who were age- and sex-matched. None of the patients had a clinical history of cardiovascular disease, nor were they diabetic or hypertensive. The two groups were comparable in living habits and body mass index. Although total fibrinolytic activity was similar for both groups, in terms of ELA, type IV patients had significantly higher t-PA antigen after venous occlusion and resting PAI-1 antigen and activity than normolipidemics. In the same study, the patients were asked to follow a dietary regimen designed to reduce TG levels for a period of 2–4 months. At the end of the dietary period, reduction in PAI-1 levels was observed only in those subjects in whom TG levels were lowered to values ≤ 2.8 mmol/L. This suggests that TG reduction toward normal levels is accompanied by a normalization in circulating PAI-1 levels.

ATHEROGENIC LIPOPROTEINS AND PAI-1 RELEASE BY ENDOTHELIAL CELLS

A number of studies indicate that atherogenic lipoproteins may interact with vascular endothelium, influencing specific properties of this protective lining and/or inducing cell cytotoxicity (16–19). Vascular endothelial cells are known to release both t-PA and PAI-1 in response to a number of pathophysiological stimuli (3). Thrombin, tumor promoters, and bacterial lipopolysaccharides are among agents that induce t-PA synthesis and release. Insulin has been shown to increase PAI-1 release by an hepatoma cell line (HepG2 cells) but not by endothelial cells (20). This effect offers a possible explanation for the increased PAI-antigen levels found in patients with hyperinsulinemia (21).

Recently, a study carried out in our laboratory demonstrated that very-low-density lipoprotein (VLDL) and low-density lipoprotein (LDL) concentrations dependently stimulate PAI-1 release by human umbilical vein endothelial cells in culture (22). The increase of PAI-1 exerted by the two different lipoprotein classes is concentration-dependent, with a maximal activity similar to that of bacterial lipopolysaccharide at the 10 μg/ml concentration. It is interesting to note that acetylation of apoB like that occurring in LDL treated with acetic anhydride—i.e., acetyl-LDL—does not reduce the capacity of lipoproteins to stimulate PAI-1 release by endothelial cells (23). In contrast, chemically oxidized LDL concentration dependently inhibit PAI-1 release. Taken together, these data, although still preliminary, suggest that atherogenic lipoproteins regulate the release of PAI-1 in a complex manner. Further work is needed to define the molecular mechanisms underlying this phenomenon.

CONCLUSIONS

The above-discussed evidence strongly suggests that increases in TG levels are associated with alterations in the fibrinolytic system, possibly resulting in an impairment of total fibrinolytic activity. Several questions, however, remain to be answered. The major question is to describe the mechanism by which TG-rich lipoproteins affect the fibrinolytic system, both at the level of PAI-1 release by competent cells and of t-PA antigen synthesis or release. Future studies of interventions either via dietary treatments or drugs known to reduce TG levels should establish whether there is a causal relationship between alterations of TG metabolism and the fibrinolytic system.

So far, *in vitro* studies indicate that both VLDL and LDL regulate PAI-1 release by endothelial cells and in some cases by hepatic cells. The available data, however, do not yet allow us to conclude that there is a causal relationship between cellular release of PAI-1, as influenced by atherogenic lipoproteins, and modifications of the fibrinolytic system in hyperlipoproteinemias. Further inquiry into the mechanisms involved in the cell-lipoprotein interaction, in terms of cellular fibrinolytic capacity, should help us to understand the alterations of the fibrinolytic system described in hyperlipoproteinemias.

REFERENCES

1. Collen D. On the regulation and control of fibrinolysis. *Thromb Haemostas* 1980;43:77–89.

2. Bachman F. Fibrinolysis. In: Verstraete M, Vermylen J, Lijnen HR, Arnout J, eds. *Thrombosis and haemostasis*. Leuven: Leuven Univ. Press, 1987;227–265.
3. Schleef RR, Loskutoff DJ. Fibrinolytic system of vascular endothelial cells. Role of plasminogen activator inhibitors. *Haemostasis* 1988;18:328–341.
4. Grieg HBW, Runde IA. Studies of the inhibition of fibrinolysis by lipids. *Lancet* 1957;2:461.
5. Hamsten A, Wiman B, de Faire U, Blomback M. Increased plasma levels of a rapid inhibitor of tissue plasminogen activator in young survivors of myocardial infarction. *N Engl J Med* 1985;313:1557–1563.
6. Juhan Vague I, Valadier J, Alessi MC, et al. Deficient t-PA release and elevated PA inhibitor levels in patients with spontaneous or recurrent deep venous thrombosis. *Thromb Haemostas* 1987;57:67–72.
7. Juhan Vague I, Roul C, Alessi MC, Ardissone JP, Helm M, P Vague. Increased plasminogen activator inhibitor activity in non–insulin dependent diabetic patients. Relationship with plasma insulin, *Thromb Haemostas* 1989;61:370–373.
8. WHO memorandum. Classification of hyperlipoproteinemias. *Circulation* 1972;45:501–508.
9. Epstein SE, Rosing DR, Brakman P, Redwood D, Astrup T. Impaired fibrinolytic response to exercise in patients with type IV hyperlipoproteinemia. *Lancet* 1970;2:631–633.
10. Cuculanu MP, Stef C, Zorenghea D, Popescu O. In vitro effect of p-chlormercuribenzoate upon dilute blood clot lysis time in hyperlipemia. *Thromb Haemostas* 1979;42:929–943.
11. Andersen P, Arnesen H, Hjermann I. Hyperlipoproteinaemia and reduced fibrinolytic activity in healthy coronary high-risk men. *Acta Medica Scandinavica* 1981;209:199–202.
12. Brommer EJP, Gevers Leuven JA, Barrett-Bregshoeff MM, Schouten JA. Response of fibrinolytic activity and factor VIII-related antigen to stimulation with desmopressin in hyperlipoproteinemia. *J Lab Clin Med* 1982;100:105–114.
13. Simpson HCR, Mann JI, Meade TW, Chakrabarti R, Sterling Y, Woolf L. Hypertriglyceridemia and hypercoagulability. *Lancet* 1983;1:786–789.
14. Oseroff A, Krishnamurti C, Hassett A, Tang D, Alving B. Plasminogen activator and plasminogen activator inhibitor activities in men with coronary artery disease. *J Lab Clin Med* 1989;113:88–93.
15. Mussoni L, Mannucci L, Sirtori M, Camera M, Maderna P, Tremoli E. Hypertriglyceridemia and regulation of fibrinolytic activity (submitted for publication).
16. Triau E, Meydani SN, Schaefer EJ. Oxidized low density lipoprotein stimulate prostacyclin production by adult human vascular endothelial cells. *Arteriosclerosis* 1988;8:810–818.
17. Kugiyama KSA, Morrisett JD, Roberts R, Henry PD. Impairment of endothelial dependent arterial relaxation by lysolecithin in modified low-density lipoproteins. *Nature* 1990;344:160–162.
18. Henriksen T, Evensen SA, Carlander B. Injury to human endothelial cells in culture induced by low density lipoproteins. *Scand J Clin Lab Invest* 1979;39:361–368.
19. Hessler JR, Robertson AL Jr, Chisolm GM. LDL-induced cytotoxicity and its inhibition by HDL in human vascular smooth muscle and endothelial cells in culture. *Atherosclerosis* 1979;32:213–229.
20. Alessi MC, Juhan Vague I, Kooistra T, deClerck F, Collen D. Insulin stimulates the synthesis of an inhibitor of tissue-type plasminogen activator inhibitor-1 by the human hepatocellular line HepG2. *Thromb Haemostas* 1988;60:491–494.
21. Juhan Vague I, Alessi MC, Joly P, et al. Plasma plasminogen activator inhibitor-1 in angina pectoris. Influence of plasma insulin and the acute phase response. *Arteriosclerosis* 1989;9:362–367.
22. Mussoni L, Maderna P, Camera M, et al. Atherogenic lipoproteins and release of plasminogen activator inhibitor-1 (PAI-1) by endothelial cells. *Fibrinolysis* 1990;4:79–81.
23. Goldstein JL, Ho YK, Basu SK, Brown MS. Binding sites on macrophages that mediates uptake and degradation of acetylated low density lipoprotein, inducing massive cholesterol deposition. *Proc Natl Acad Sci USA* 1979;76:333–337.

Atherosclerosis Reviews, Volume 22,
edited by A. M. Gotto, Jr. and R. Paoletti.
Raven Press, Ltd., New York © 1991.

Interrelation of Lp(a) with Plasma Triglycerides

Gert M. Kostner

Institute of Medical Biochemistry, University of Graz, A-8010 Graz, Austria

Lp(a) is an apolipoprotein B (apoB)-containing lipoprotein of human plasma that resembles low-density lipoprotein (LDL) in chemical composition and morphology [for a review, see ref. 1]. In fact, Lp(a) may be best described as an LDL particle with an additional protein, apo-a, attached to it, probably via one disulfid bridge. Research interest in Lp(a) has been growing expo-nentionálly in the last few years because (a) this lipoprotein seems to be one of the most atherogenic fractions in plasma, and (b) the structure of apo-a is highly homologous to plasminogen. Thus, it may represent the missing link between the pathophysiology of hemostasis and that of lipid metabolism (2,3).

Despite the structural similarity of Lp(a) and LDL, these two lipoproteins metabolize quite differently. Although Lp(a) competes for LDL binding to the B/E receptor in *in vitro* experiments, there are some indications that Lp(a) might not be catabolized via this route *in vivo,* since lipid-lowering drugs that effectively increase the number of B/E R-receptors in the liver barely influence plasma Lp(a) levels (4). In *in vivo* experiments in humans, we have shown that triglyceride-rich lipoproteins (TGRLP) are not the pre-cursor of Lp(a). We therefore postulated that Lp(a) is produced directly by the liver and secreted into the bloodstream (5).

We still know very little about the relationship between plasma TG me-tabolism and Lp(a). In early experiments dating back to 1983, we found that type IV hyperlipemics do not run an increased risk for atherosclerosis if they have high plasma Lp(a) levels (6). In fact, statistical evaluations have indicated that Lp(a) in this subgroup even protects the individual to some extent. To pursue this issue further, we set out to investigate the interaction of TG-rich particles with Lp(a).

MATERIALS AND METHODS

Lp(a) from strongly Lp(a)-positive individuals was purified by ultracen-triugation at d = 1.070–1.120, followed by Biogel A-5m column chromatography (3,4). Purity and chemical integrity were assessed by immunochemical methods and polyacrylamide gel electrophoresis. Chemical analyses were performed according to standard laboratory procedures (5,6). Lipofundin was purchased from Braun-Melsungen (F.R.G.).

RESULTS

Lp(a) as a Risk Factor for Atherosclerosis

Table 1 gives the Lp(a) values of post-myocardial infarction (MI) individuals in relation to controls. The groups are subdivided into patients with different forms of hyperlipoproteinemia. The normolipemics were individuals with plasma TG < 160 mg/dl and cholesterol values of < 260 mg/dl. Assuming a cut-off level for Lp(a) of 30 mg/dl, the relative risk for MI in the normolipemic group was 1.75. In the group of type IIa individuals, it was 6.5; and for type IIb hyperlipemics, it was 2.3. Only the type IV individuals were different. There were twice as many Lp(a)-positive individuals in the control group as compared to the MI group. From these results, we conclude that Lp(a) is not a risk factor in type IV individuals.

Distribution of Apo-A Among Various Density Fractions

Conflicting results have been published with respect to the distribution of the Lp(a) antigen within the plasma lipoprotein spectrum (7,8). After studying this issue in detail using ultracentrifugation, polyanion precipitation, and immunochemical methods (9), we found that in fasting plasma, ~ 95% of

TABLE 1. *Lp(a) plasma concentration in post-myocardial infarction individuals in comparison to controls*

	% of Individuals		
Type of patients	Lp(a) <30 mg/dl	Lp(a) >30 mg/dl	Relative risk
Normolipemics[a]			
Controls	74.5	25.5	
MI	55.5	44.5	1.75
Type IIA			
Controls	87.6	12.4	
MI	19.5	80.5	6.5
Type IIB			
Controls	79.0	21.0	
MI	51.7	48.3	2.3
Type IV			
Controls	67.4	32.6	
MI	84.5	15.5	—2.1

[a] Cut-off levels: TG <160 mg/dl; TC <260 mg/dl.

the Lp(a) immune reactivity was present in the HDL_2 density class. The rest was found almost exclusively in the d = 1.21 bottom. Whether or not this latter fraction was attached to apoB or lipids could not be assessed unequivocally.

Lp(a) in Postprandial Plasma

It has been suggested previously that apo-a immune reactivity is also present in d < 1.006 lipoproteins, notably in chylomicrons (CYM) and their remnants (10). We have also detected apo-a in TGRLP using Western blotting, but by this method the actual fraction of apo-a in d < 1.006 lipoproteins cannot be measured. We therefore studied apo-a in the postprandial phase by Laurell electrophoresis in the bottom fraction after removal of CYM and large remnants by ultracentrifugation at d 1.006 g/ml.

The results (Table 2) demonstrate that apo-a immune reactivity in the d = 1.006 bottom decreases 4 hr to 8 hr postprandially, but it reaches the original fasting values again after 24 hr. It is noteworthy that the maximal decrease of Lp(a) in the postprandial phase amounts to ~ 5%, which is actually the value of free apo-a present in the lipoprotein free-bottom fraction. We have not investigated whether or not there was any free apo-a left 4 hr to 6 hr postprandially, but our observations are compatible with the assumption that total apo-a in plasma is not affected by the fatty meal, and there is a shift of the free apo-a portion toward the TG-rich d < 1.006 fraction.

Influence of Intravenously Infused Lipid Plasma Lp(a)

There are several artificial lipid emulsions for intravenous therapy on the market that differ in TG concentration, kind of emulsifier, and size of the lipid droplets. Although we have studied several of them, reported here are only the results obtained with Lipofundin (Braun-Melsungen).

TABLE 2. *Distribution of Lp(a) immune reactivity in the d > 1.006 g/ml fraction in comparison to total plasma after a fatty meal*

Initials	Hr after the fat meal				
	0	4	8	12	24
S.P.	100	97	95	99	102
F.S.	100	93	94	98	105
A.F.	100	95	94	97	103

Three volunteers were given a triglyceride-rich diet corresponding to 1 g TG per kg of body weight. The Lp(a) distribution in the density > and < 1.006 g/ml was measured by Laurell electrophoresis. Lp(a) plasma concentrations varied between 12 and 42 mg/dl. The values are given in percentage of Lp(a) immune reactivity found in the d > 1.006 bottom fraction.

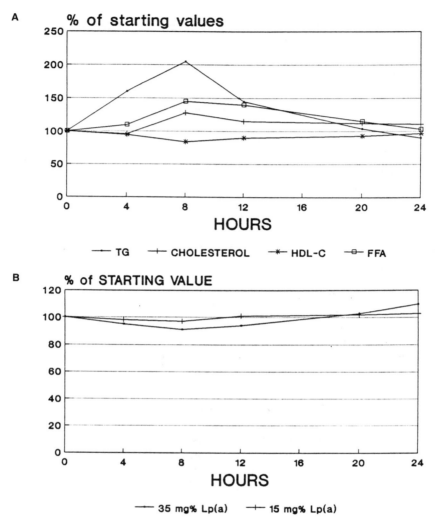

FIG. 1. **(A)** Two normolipemic healthy male volunteers with 15 and 35 mg/dl of Lp(a), respectively, were infused with Lipofundin 0.1 g/kg body weight/hr for 8 hr, and their plasma lipids and lipoproteins were analyzed at the given intervals. The values are means, given in percentage of the zero starting hour. **(B)** The same experiment as (A), but the values represent fluctuations of plasma Lp(a) levels of the two individuals.

Two volunteers with fasting Lp(a) levels of 15 and 35 mg/dl were infused intravenously for 8 hr with 0.1 g TG/kg body weight per hr and their plasma lipid and Lp(a) levels were followed for 24 hr. The results are shown in Fig. 1. As expected, TG values increased by ~ 100% and cholesterol values increased by ~ 10% during the first 8 hr of the experiment. HDL cholesterol values decreased by some 15%. Concerning Lp(a) immune reactivity, one proband reacted with an ~ 5% to 10% decrease during the first 8 hr, followed by an increase thereafter. The 24-hr value of this proband was ~ 5% higher than the starting value. The Lp(a) values of the other proband remained virtually unchanged during the 24-hr observation period.

We conclude from these experiments that there is no interrelationship of Lp(a) with TG metabolism. Lp(a) is not derived from normal very-low-density lipoproteins (VLDL) secreted by the liver. Chylomicrons by themselves must also be excluded as precursors, since no B-48 is found in Lp(a). Chylomicrons, on the other hand, may serve as an acceptor of free apo-a, which is present in fasting plasma in amounts of 4% to 5% of total Lp(a). During clearance of CYM by the lipoprotein lipase, this "adsorbed" apo-a appears to remain in circulation. Whether or not this feature has any physiological significance on one hand, or whether it is linked to the pronounced atherogenicity of Lp(a) on the other, is yet to be determined.

ACKNOWLEDGMENTS

This study was supported by grants from the Austrian National Bank (grant no. 3382) and the Austrian Research Foundation, Programme Project S-46 (principal investigator, G.M.K.).

REFERENCES

1. Kostner GM. Lp(a) lipoproteins and the genetic polymorphisms of lipoprotein B. In: Day CE, Levy RS, eds. *Low density lipoproteins.* New York: Plenum Press, 1976:229–269.
2. McLean JW, Tomlinson JE, Kuang WJ, et al. cDNA sequence of human apolipoprotein(a) is homologous to plasminogen. *Nature* 1987;300:132–137.
3. Karadi I, Kostner GM, Gries A, et al. Lipoprotein (a) and plasminogen are immunochemically related. *Biochim Biophys Acta* 1988;960:91–97.
4. Kostner GM, Gavish D, Leopold B, et al. HMG-CoA reductase inhibitors lower LDL but increase Lp(a) levels. A study of 24 individuals treated with Simvastatin or Lovastatin. *Circulation* 1989;80:1313–1319.
5. Krempler F, Kostner GM, Bolzano K, Sandhofer F. Lipoprotein (a) is not a metabolic product of other lipoproteins containing apolipoprotein B. *Biochim Biophys Acta* 1979;575:63–70.
6. Kostner GM, Avogaro P, Cazzolato G, et al. Lipoprotein Lp(a) and the risk for myocardial infarction. *Atherosclerosis* 1981;38:51–61.
7. Fless GM, ZumMallen ME, Scanu AM. Physicochemical properties of apo-a and lipoprotein (a–) derived from dissociation of human plasma Lp(a). *J Biol Chem* 1986;261:8712–8718.
8. Utermann G. The mysteries of lipoprotein (a). *Science* 1989;246:904–910.
9. Gries A, Nimpf J, Nimpf M, et al. Free and apo-B associated Lpa-specific protein in human serum. *Clin Chim Acta* 1987;164:93–100.
10. Gaubatz JW, Chari MV, Nava ML, et al. Isolation and characterization of two major apolipoproteins in human lipoprotein-a. *J Lipid Res* 1987;28:69–79.

Atherosclerosis Reviews, Volume 22,
edited by A. M. Gotto, Jr. and R. Paoletti.
Raven Press, Ltd., New York © 1991.

Plasma Lp(a) Patterns After Triglyceride Infusion

M. Rosseneu, C. Labeur, N. Vinaimont, *J. P. De Slypere, and †E. Matthys

*Department of Clinical Biochemistry, A.Z. St-Jan, Brugge; *Department of Endocrinology, University Hospital, Gent; and †Department of Nephrology, A.Z. St-Jan, Brugge, Belgium*

The Lp(a) lipoprotein represents an additional and independent risk factor for the development of coronary heart disease (1), although the mechanism through which Lp(a) accelerates the development of atherosclerotic lesions has not been elucidated yet.

The accumulation of Lp(a) in atherosclerotic plaques might be due to its interaction with proteoglycans (2). Bersot et al (3) have suggested that the enrichment of β-very-low-density lipoproteins (VLDL) and chylomicra-remnants with Lp(a), after a fat-rich meal, might enhance the uptake of these lipoproteins through the scavenger receptor and lead to increased foam cell formation. Recent data (4) suggest that the low-density lipoproteins (LDL) receptor might be involved in Lp(a) catabolism as plasma Lp(a) levels are increased in patients with familial hypercholesterolemia and defective receptor activity (5). Further hypothesis include a competition of Lp(a) for binding to the tissue plasminogen receptor and impairment of fibrinolysis (6).

In plasma, Lp(a) appears as a distinct lipoprotein fraction, consisting of apoB, apo(a), and lipids, with a size and density intermediate between those of LDL and high-density lipoproteins (HDL). It has been shown however, that Lp(a) can redistribute towards triglyceride-rich lipoproteins (TRLP) after fat ingestion.

The metabolic fate and the clearance of the Lp(a) fractions are still unresolved. For this purpose we examined the distribution of Lp(a) between Lp(a) fraction in the normal density range (i.e., 1.05–1.10 g/ml), and TRLP in normolipemic individuals and in patients with impaired renal function. These data should provide information about the transfer mechanism of Lp(a) between lipoproteins and about their possible routes of catabolism.

MATERIALS AND METHODS

Subjects

An intralipid infusion was administered to three normolipidemic volunteers, to one patient with a nephrotic syndrome and to one patient with impaired renal function treated by continuous ambulatory peritoneal dialysis (CAPD). The lipids and apolipoproteins of the five individuals before intralipid infusion are listed in Table 1.

Study Protocol

An infusion of 350 ml/2.5 m² of a 20% intralipid emulsion (Kabi Vitrum, Stockholm, Sweden) was administered to the five volunteers for a period of 2.5 hr. Blood was drawn on EDTA before and at 30 min, 1, 2, 3, 4, 5 or 6, 8, and 24 hr after beginning the infusion. The volunteers consumed only beverages during that period. Plasma lipids and apolipoproteins including cholesterol, triglycerides (TG), phospholipids, apoA-I, B, C-II, C-III, A-IV, and Lp(a) were measured at the various time intervals by methods previously described (7).

Lipoprotein fractions were separated by gel filtration from 0.2 ml plasma applied to a Superose 6HR column (8). TRLP, LDL, the Lp(a) fraction, and HDL could be resolved after quantitation of the appropriate apolipoproteins in the various fractions of the eluate (8). These separations were carried out on samples collected at 0, 0.5, 2, 5 or 6 and 24 hr after beginning the infusion. The percentages of Lp(a) and the other apolipoproteins in the different lipoprotein fractions were calculated.

The Lp(a) phenotypes were determined after separation of the apo(a)

TABLE 1. *Plasma lipids and apolipoproteins (mg/dl) after triglyceride infusion*

Patient	Hr	TG	Chol	PL	ApoA-I	ApoB	ApoC-III	Lp(a)	Lp(a) phen
V.D.P.	0	137	241	232	133	100	14.8	84	S2
	2	673	282	407	105	88	10.9	67	
J.J.	0	104	200	201	166	71	19.1	45	S2/S4
	2	627	254	383	150	68	15.5	41	
O.F.	0	255	250	242	116	98	22.2	48	S3
	2	462	286	309	113	88	18.6	33	
C.G.	0	191	297	227	148	159	37.6	235	S1
	2	509	301	282	98	103	34.1	198	
	8	487	267	267	95	93	35.2	150	
M.J.	0	400	242	237	75	140	35.3	52	S3/S4
	3	970	299	350	84	124	33.3	35	

TG, triglyceride; chol, cholesterol; PL, phospholipids; Hr, hours; phen, phenotype.

isoforms by SDS polyacrylamide gel electrophoresis in 6% acrylamide gels and blotting of the fractions onto nitrocellulose. Detection was performed using a polyclonal antiserum against Lp(a) which had been affinity purified to eliminate anti-apoB cross-reactivity.

RESULTS

Plasma Lipid and Apolipoprotein Concentrations After TG Infusion

The plasma triglycerides, cholesterol, and phospholipids measured at the intervals stated above are depicted in Fig. 1B for a normolipemic subject and Fig. 1A in a CAPD patient. In both subjects, a maximum of the TG

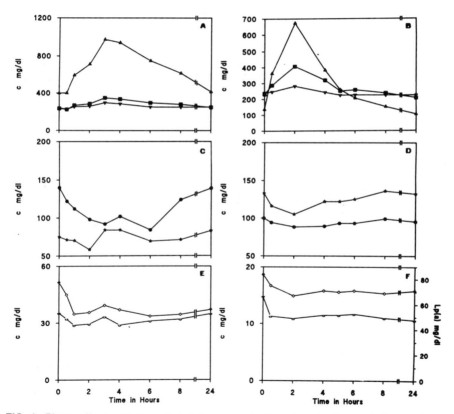

FIG. 1. Plasma lipid and apolipoprotein concentrations in volunteers, during and after administration of an Intralipid infusion. Triglycerides (▲), cholesterol (▼) and phospholipids (■), apoA-I (★), apoB (●), apoC-III (▽), Lp(a) (◇). (**A,C,E**) CAPD patients, (**B,D,F**): normolipemic volunteers.

concentration was reached after 3 hr to 4 hr, followed by a subsequent decrease of the plasma concentrations until the basal level was reached again after 8 hr to 24 hr. Although the increases were less pronounced, the same pattern was observed for the phospholipid and cholesterol levels.

The variation in the apoA-I and B concentrations was dependent upon the individual treated. At first, the apoA-I and B concentrations decreased in most patients (Fig. 1C), but returned to their original values after 2 hr to 4 hr. The decrease was less pronounced in the normolipemic volunteers (Fig. 1D).

For the apoC-III and apoA-IV patterns, we observed a slight decrease in concentration at the onset of the infusion, followed by a stabilization of the concentration at a level either equal or slightly lower than the original value (Fig. 1E and F).

As with the apoC-III, the Lp(a) concentration decreased slightly and further stabilized after 2 hr to 4 hr after beginning the infusion (Fig. 1E and F).

Lp(a) Distribution in the Lipoprotein Fractions

After separation of the plasma lipoproteins by gel filtration, Lp(a) was assayed in the TGRLP and in the Lp(a) fraction in two normolipemic patients

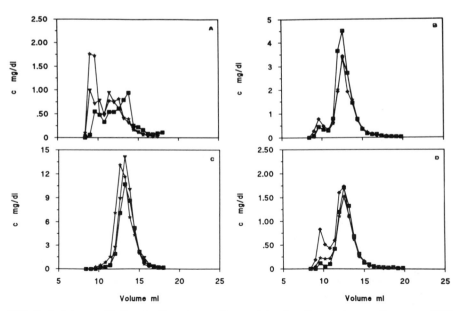

FIG. 2. Lp(a) quantitation in the plasma lipoproteins fractionated on a Superose 6HR column during Intralipid infusion. (**A**) CAPD patient, (**B**) patient with a nephrotic syndrome; (**C,D**) normolipemic volunteers. Sampling times are (■) 0 hr; (∇) 2 hr; (◆) 5 hr; (*) 24 hr.

(Fig. 2B and D), in the CAPD patient (Fig. 2A) and in the patient with a nephrotic syndrome (Fig. 2C). We observed a transfer of Lp(a) from the Lp(a) fraction located between LDL and HDL toward the TGRLP. This effect is maximal at 4 hr to 6 hr. The magnitude of the transfer depends on the individual (Fig.2).

From these data we calculated both the amount and relative percentage of Lp(a) in the Lp(a) fraction and in the TRLP as a function of the sampling time (Fig. 3). In all subjects, we observed a decreased concentration of the Lp(a) fraction at the normal density and an increase of the Lp(a) content of the TRLP, with a maximal effect at 2 hr to 5 hr. The percentages of Lp(a) in the TG-rich fraction vary strongly between individuals, from < 10% in one patient, although the plasma Lp(a) concentration was 250 mg/dl, up to ~ 50% for the CAPD patient (Table 2).

We examined the phenotype distribution in plasma, in the Lp(a) fraction, and in the TGRLP of the heterozygote volunteers with phenotypes S2/4 and S3/4. In both patients, we clearly observed a preferential transfer of the largest isoform (S4 phenotype) toward the TGRLP (data not shown).

TABLE 2. *Distribution of Lp(a) in triglyceride-rich lipoprotein (TGRLP) and Lp(a) fraction after triglyceride infusion*

Patient	Time (hr)	TGRLP Lp(a) (%)	Lp(a) fraction (%)
V.D.P.	0	7.6	92.4
	0.5	9.1	90.9
	2	9.3	90.7
	5	15.3	84.7
	24	8.5	91.5
J.J.	0	4.3	95.7
	0.5	4.8	95.2
	2	16.4	83.6
	5	25.6	74.4
	24	12.1	87.9
O.F.	0	18.0	82.0
	0.5	12.2	87.8
	2	16.9	83.1
	6	14.8	85.2
	24	20.9	79.1
C.G.	0	1.4	98.6
	0.5	1.8	98.2
	2	1.0	99.0
	6	4.2	95.8
	24	3.2	96.8
M.J.	0	26.9	73.1
	0.5	21.3	78.7
	2	53.5	46.5
	6	50.2	49.8
	24	61.0	39.0

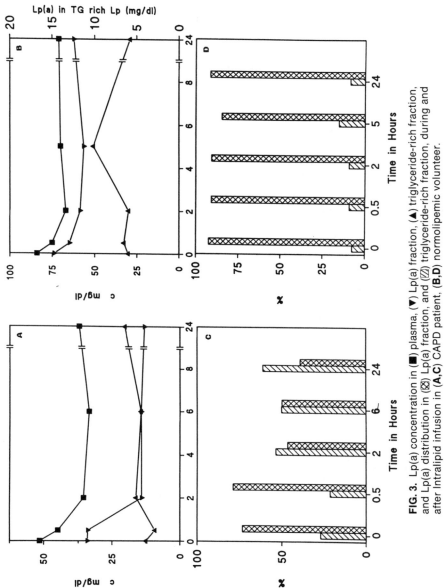

FIG. 3. Lp(a) concentration in (■) plasma, (▼) Lp(a) fraction, (▲) triglyceride-rich fraction, and Lp(a) distribution in (⊠) Lp(a) fraction, and (▨) triglyceride-rich fraction, during and after Intralipid infusion in (**A,C**) CAPD patient, (**B,D**) normolipemic volunteer.

CONCLUSION

The administration of a TG infusion to normolipemic volunteers and to patients with impaired renal function enabled the study of the interaction of Lp(a) with TGRLP. During and after the infusion, we observed a significant transfer of Lp(a) toward the TG-rich fractions. The largest Lp(a) isoform appears to be transfered preferentially. This process was accompanied by a decreased concentration of the Lp(a) fraction, resulting in a significant increase in the percentage of Lp(a) in the TG-rich fraction. This effect was strongly dependent on the individual and not correlated to the plasma Lp(a) concentration.

The mechanism of disappearance of Lp(a) from the TGRLP, i.e., whether it either receptor-mediated or not, still remains a topic for further investigation.

REFERENCES

1. Sandkamp M, Funke H, Schulte H, Köhler E, Assman G. Lipoprotein (a) is an independent risk factor for myocardial infarction at a young age. *Clin Chem* 1990;36:20–23.
2. Bihari-Varga M, Gruber E, Rotheneder M, Zechner R, Kostner G. Interaction of lipoprotein Lp(a) and low density lipoprotein with glycaminoglycans from human aorta. *Arteriosclerosis* 1988;8:851–857.
3. Bersot T, Innerarity T, Pitas R, Rall S, Weisgraber K, Mahley R. Fat feeding in humans induces lipoproteins of density less than 1.006 that are enriched in apolipoprotein (a) and that cause lipid accumulation in macrophages. *J Clin Invest* 1989;77:622–630.
4. Utermann G. The mysteries of lipoprotein (a). *Science* 1989;246:904–910.
5. Utermann G, Hopplicher F, Dieplinger H, Seed M, Thompson G, Boerwinkel E. Defects in the low density lipoprotein receptor gene affect lipoproteins Lp(a) levels: multiplicative interaction of two gene loci associated with premature atherosclerosis. *Proc Natl Acad Sci USA* 1989;86:4171–4174.
6. Miles L, Fless GM, Levin EG, Scanu AM, Plox EF. A potential basis for the thrombotic risks myocardial infarction at a young age. *Nature* 1989;339:301–302.
7. Labeur C, Shepherd J, Rosseneu M. Lipoprotein (a) quantified by an enzyme linked immunosorbent assay with monoclonal antibodies. *Clin Chem* 1990;36:591–597.
8. Van Biervliet JP, Labeur C, Michiels G, Usher DC, Rosseneu M. Lipoprotein profiles and evolution in newborns. *Atherosclerosis* 1991;86:173–181.

Atherosclerosis Reviews, Volume 22,
edited by A. M. Gotto, Jr. and R. Paoletti.
Raven Press, Ltd., New York © 1991.

Diet in the Treatment of Hypertriglyceridemia

P. J. Nestel

Division of Human Nutrition, Commonwealth Scientific and Industrial Organization, Adelaide, South Australia 5000, Australia

Hypertriglyceridemia comprises a group of abnormal lipoprotein phenotypes. The familial forms include:

solitary chylomicronemia,
solitary hypertriglyceridemia,
hypertriglyceridemia + low high-density lipoprotein (HDL),
hypertriglyceridemia + hyperapobetalipoproteinemia,
combined hyperlipoproteinemia, and apoE-related dyslipoproteinemia.

All these forms are affected by such environmental factors as excess energy, leading to obesity, and alcohol. These factors may change the phenotype. Because all these hyperlipidemias stem from different metabolic disturbances, standard dietary treatment is not uniformly successful. Often, triglyceride (TG) [in very-low-density lipoproteins (VLDL)] is reduced, but cholesterol [in low-density lipoproteins (LDL)] rises; and low HDL levels may not rise. Furthermore, plasma TG levels can fluctuate substantially in these disorders.

Because it is a risk for pancreatitis and not for atherosclerosis, solitary chylomicronemia will not be considered here. A very low fat intake in which fat energy is provided by medium-chain TG reduces TG levels to below-risk threshold.

The need to treat milder forms of hypertriglyceridemia is determined by the likely risk for atherosclerosis. This rule of thumb is used whether raised TG is part of a complex hyperlipidemia or whether it is associated with other non-lipid risk factors. Less certain is the decision to treat when hypertriglyceridemia is modest and represents the sole atherogenic factor; however, it is reasonable to attend to the diet if the cause is excess alcohol or obesity, which is often the case. More difficult is the question of risk when mild hypertriglyceridemia is associated with low HDL but normal—or even low—LDL. This condition is common in Third World countries, due to the low-fat, high-carbohydrate diets of their peoples. However, such a diet gives rise to a similar lipid pattern in affluent societies. Epidemiologists regard any reduction in HDL as a potential risk, yet many nutritionists would not intervene.

Excess energy, regardless of the mix of nutrients in the diet, may cause hypertriglyceridemia. Overweight causes many disturbances in lipid metabolism, including TG overproduction [partly due to a high free fatty acid (FFA) turnover] and diminished TG removal (especially if resistance to insulin develops). Normal weight is a prerequisite for normal TG levels.

An excess of carbohydrates in the diet has traditionally been regarded as a common cause of hypertriglyceridemia. However, classic severe carbohydrate-induced hypertriglyceridemia is rare. To what extent, then, does carbohydrate intake matter? In our experience, problems occur only in the context of unusually high intakes (1,2). In some individuals, it may account for highly variable TG levels. When carbohydrate intake $> 60\%$ energy (and fat falls to $< 25\%$ energy), the sucrose/starch ratio becomes important. At more usual intakes, sucrose does not raise TG more than starch, nor is eating fructose worse than glucose. Hypertriglyceridemic subjects are more susceptible to sudden changes in energy intake than normal people. Triglyceride levels can rise steeply after a few days of overeating (1). Carbohydrate-rich diets stimulate VLDL secretion (2), but they also increase LDL apoB and HDL apoA-1 clearance.

Alcohol is another common source of sudden variability in TG levels. VLDL triglyceride secretion rises within hours and is much greater in hypertriglyceridemic than normal subjects (3). Because the clearance of chylomicron remnants is reduced by alcohol, alcohol taken with fatty meals is particularly hypertriglyceridemic.

The nature of dietary fatty acids had not been regarded as important until the introduction of the n-3 fatty acids from fish. These FA are highly potent TG-lowering nutrients; reductions of up to 50% are common with high dosage. Furthermore, they are effective even in the complex hyperlipidemias, except for isolated chylomicronemia. We have recently shown that only the marine n-3 fatty acids are effective, not α-linolenic acid (the major plant n-3 fatty acid) (4).

Marine n-3 fatty acids influence triglyceride metabolism profoundly. Some of the mechanisms are reduced TG synthesis, reduced VLDL secretion and turnover, diminished esterifying enzyme activities, diminished fatty acid synthesis, and increased fatty acid oxidation. Although the two major FA, eicosapentaenoic (EPA) and docosahexaenoic (DHA), do not act identically, in clinical practice the plasma TG-lowering effects are similar.

However, the effect of n-3 fatty acids on other lipoproteins can be unpredictable. Recent reports (5,6) have documented the fact that LDL cholesterol levels may rise. Although the increase is particularly likely in cases of isolated hypertriglyceridemia, it is also seen in the complex hyperlipidemias. In combined hyperlipoproteinemia, LDL cholesterol and LDL apoB may be differentially affected, so that the overall change in lipoprotein phenotype may deteriorate (despite lowered VLDL). It is not known whether the effects are the same for both EPA and DHA, or whether other constituents in the oils are the cause. Of the other common nutrients, neither fiber nor protein has an important effect on TG concentration.

An additional reason for treating hypertriglyceridemia is its association with thrombogenic factors. Although the mechanism is unclear, there is a strong correlation between fat intake and circulating coagulant factors (7).

Thus, dietary treatment of hypertriglyceridemia is the obvious solution when the cause is excess energy or alcohol. Managing hyperlipidemias that are primarily genetic in origin can be difficult. Although fish oil fatty acids do normalize TG levels, the overall effect on the lipoprotein phenotype may be less than optimal.

REFERENCES

1. Nestel PJ, Carroll KF, Havenstein N. Plasma triglyceride response to carbohydrates, fats and caloric intake. *Metabolism* 1970;19:1–18.
2. Huff MW, Nestel PJ. Metabolism of apolipoproteins CII, CIII$_1$, CIII$_2$ and VLDL-B in human subjects consuming high carbohydrate diets. *Metabolism* 1982;31:493–498.
3. Taskinen M-R, Nikkila EA. Nocturnal hypertriglyceridemia and hyperinsulinemia following moderate evening intake of alcohol. *Acta Med Scand* 1977;202:172–177.
4. Kestin M, Clifton P, Belling GB, Nestel PJ. N-3 fatty acids of marine origin lower systolic blood pressure and triglycerides but raise LDL cholesterol compared with n-3 and n-6 fatty acids from plants. *Am J Clin Nutr* 1990;1:1028–1034.
5. Harris WS. Fish oils and plasma lipid and lipoprotein metabolism in humans: a critical review. *J Lipid Res* 1989;30:785–808.
6. Nestel PJ. Effects of n-3 fatty acids on lipid metabolism. *Annu Rev Nutr* 1990;10:149–167.
7. Miller GJ, Cruickshank JK, Ellis LJ, et al. Fat consumption and factor VII coagulant activity in middle-aged men. *Atherosclerosis* 1989;78:19–24.

Atherosclerosis Reviews, Volume 22,
edited by A. M. Gotto, Jr. and R. Paoletti.
Raven Press, Ltd., New York © 1991.

Effect of Bile Acid Sequestrants on Triglyceride Metabolism

Sverker Ericsson and Bo Angelin

Metabolism Unit, Department of Medicine, Karolinska Institute at Huddinge University Hospital, S-141 86 Huddinge, Sweden

Bile acid sequestrants are potent lipid-lowering drugs that effectively lower low-density lipoprotein (LDL) cholesterol and thereby reduce the risk for development of ischemic heart disease (1,2).

By trapping bile acids—particularly the dihydroxy ones—in the gut, these compounds promote the excretion of bile acids to the feces (3). This increased fecal loss of bile acids releases the product inhibition of bile acid formation in the hepatocyte and thus stimulates bile acid synthesis (4). This in turn enhances the demand for cholesterol in the liver cell, resulting in an induced endogenous sterol production—by stimulation of HMG CoA reductase activity—and a parallel increase in the LDL receptor expression, leading to a lowering of plasma LDL levels (5,6). In humans, treatment with 16 g of cholestyramine daily activates the cholesterol 7 α-hydroxylase (rate-determining step in bile acid production) about sixfold (7) and the HMG CoA reductase about fivefold (5), while the LDL receptor expression is increased two- to threefold (5).

Several lines of evidence demonstrate that the metabolism of triglycerides (TG) is related to the metabolism of bile acids in humans. Thus, induction of an enhanced bile acid formation with cholestyramine treatment or biliary drainage is associated with an increased production rate of TG (8,9). Furthermore, suppression of bile acid synthesis with chenodeoxycholic acid results in a reduction of plasma TG synthesis (8). Apparently, the enterohepatic circulation of bile acids might be of regulatory importance for the biosynthesis of TG in the liver.

EFFECTS ON PLASMA LIPOPROTEIN METABOLISM

The increased expression of hepatic LDL receptor activity during treatment with cholestyramine is reflected in a higher fractional catabolic rate of LDL in both hypercholesterolemic and normolipidemic subjects (2,10). As a consequence, the plasma level of LDL cholesterol may be reduced by

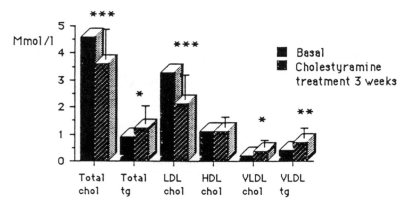

FIG. 1. Plasma lipoprotein profile in nine healthy male subjects during basal conditions and after 3 weeks of cholestyramine treatment in a daily dose of 8 g b.i.d. *$p < 0.05$; **$p < 0.05$; ***$p < 0.001$.

as much as 20% to 25% (2,10). This decrease is often associated with raised plasma levels of very-low-density lipoprotein (VLDL) TG and cholesterol (Fig. 1). Witztum et al. (11) have reported that the composition and size of VLDL particles of normotriglyceridemic subjects changed during the first month of colestipol treatment, with a transient increase in TG concentration and particle size. Similar results were obtained by our group in a recent study of familial cholesterolemia (FH) patients (12), where the VLDL TG kinetics was measured by the [³H] glycerol technique and the size of the VLDL particles was determined by electron microscopy. After 5 to 7 weeks of treatment with cholestyramine, 16 g daily, the VLDL TG levels increased by 50%, secondary to an enhanced production rate of the lipoprotein by 85%. This increase was, however, counteracted by an enhanced fractional catabolic rate of VLDL TG (by ≈ 40%). Electron micrographs of the isolated VLDL particles revealed that the lipoproteins enlarged by ~ 20% during the 1st week of treatment, but normalized after 5 to 7 weeks. Apparently, the induced catabolism of the VLDL particles thus compensates for the initial effect of an increased production of enlarged particles.

We can only speculate on the mechanisms underlying these events (Fig. 2). The increased production of VLDL must, however, be secondary to the changes in bile acid enterophepatic circulation. The secondary activation of the HMG CoA reductase, in order to provide cholesterol for the induced bile acid synthesis, may also "channel" some of the cholesterol to VLDL formation and thus stimulate the production of these lipoproteins. The TG reduction observed in response to the institution of HMG CoA inhibitors during cholestyramine therapy (13) supports this concept of a role for HMG COA reductase also in TG and VLDL metabolism.

Another potentially important mechanism for these alterations in TG me-

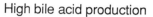

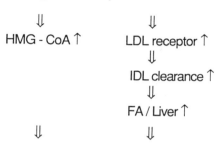

FIG. 2. Postulated mechanisms by which VLDL production increases in response to bile acid malabsorption.

tabolism may be the induced LDL receptor expression during cholestyramine therapy (14). The induction of these receptors leads to an increased uptake not only of LDL but also of VLDL remnant particles and intermediate-density lipoproteins (IDL). The increased influx of TG-rich particles into the hepatocytes enrich these cells with fatty acids; this process may also trigger VLDL synthesis. In the rat, stimulation of bile acid formation by a biliary fistula or with cholestyramine treatment increased the activity of phosphatidic acid phosphatase (PAP) about 100% and 70%, respectively (15). This enzyme could be a key regulatory step in TG biosynthesis and may thus represent a link between bile acid and TG metabolism. However, no conclusive data are yet available on the situation in humans.

The stimulated clearance of VLDL particles is also poorly understood at present. An increased LDL receptor activity may contribute to this phenomenon, but other factors, such as an increase in lipoprotein lipase action, may also be present. In other situations where VLDL TG production is stimulated, such as carbohydrate-feeding (16) or obesity (17), a similar situation with increased TG influx is also balanced by stimulated catabolism, presumably due to increased lipoprotein lipase activity. The changes in VLDL particle size distribution observed (12) indirectly lend support to the view that such an adaptive mechanism would take more than a week to fully compensate for the increased rate of synthesis induced by cholestyramine.

BILE ACIDS AND HYPERTRIGLYCERIDEMIA

The finding that considerable compensatory VLDL TG clearance can normally occur when VLDL production is augmented by the interruption of bile acid enterohepatic circulation may also be of interest when considering the pathogenesis of familial hypertriglyceridemia. In this condition, bile acid overproduction appears to represent an early stage in the development of disease—it is demonstrable before the development of manifest hypertriglyceridemia (18). Evidence from turnover studies with autologous and homologous LDL indicates that some patients with hypertriglyceridemia also show increased expression of hepatic LDL receptors (19). It may therefore be speculated that—in at least some forms of familial hypertriglyceridemia—the enhanced VLDL production caused by bile acid malabsorption is frequently compensated for by stimulation of catabolism. However, when the elimination capacity is overloaded, as may occur with increasing age (20) or weight gain (17), VLDL TG levels become elevated.

Obviously, the mechanisms by which TG metabolism is altered with resin treatment or bile acid malabsorption are still not completely understood. However, several lines of evidence indicate that this effect is mediated via the activation of the HMG CoA reductase or the induced LDL receptor activity. Also the PAP enzyme represents an attractive possibility as a key regulatory step in this respect. Ongoing studies are clarifying the role of this enzyme in bile acid metabolism.

ACKNOWLEDGMENTS

This research was supported by the Swedish Medical Research Council (03X-7137) and the King Gustaf V and Queen Victoria Foundation. We thank Ms. Lena Ericsson for manuscript preparation.

REFERENCES

1. Lipid Research Clinics Program. The Lipid Research Clinics Primary Prevention Trial Results. I. Reduction in incidence of coronary heart disease. *JAMA* 1984;251:351–364.
2. Shepherd J, Packard CJ, Bicker S, Lawrie TD, Morgan HG. Cholestyramine promotes receptor-mediated low-density lipoprotein catabolism. *N Engl J Med* 1980;302:1219–1222.
3. Thale M, Faergeman O. Binding of bile acids to anion exchanging drugs in vitro. *Scand J Gastroenterol.* 1978;13:353–356.
4. Andersén E. The effect of cholestyramine on bile acid kinetics in healthy controls. *Scand J Gastroenterol* 1979;14:657–662.
5. Reihnér E, Angelin B, Rudling M, Ewerth S, Björkhem I, Einarsson K. Regulation of hepatic cholesterol metabolism in man: stimulatory effects of cholestyramine on HMG CoA reductase activity and low density lipoprotein receptor expression in gallstone patients. *J Lipid Res* 1990;31:2219–2226.
6. Angelin B, Einarsson K. Regulation of HMG CoA reductase in human liver. In: Preiss B, ed. *Regulation of HMG CoA reductase.* New York: Academic Press, 1985:281–320.
7. Reihnér E, Björkhem I, Angelin B, Ewerth S, Einarsson K. Bile acid synthesis in humans: regulation of hepatic microsomal cholesterol 7 α-hydroxylase activity. *Gastroenterology* 1989;97:1498–1505.
8. Angelin B, Einarsson K, Hellström K, Leijd B. Effects of cholestyramine and chenodeoxycholic acid on the metabolism of endogenous triglyceride in hyperlipoproteinemia. *J Lipid Res* 1978;19:1017–1024.
9. Nestel PJ, Grundy SM. Changes in plasma triglyceride metabolism during withdrawal of bile. *Metabolism* 1976;25:1259–1268.
10. Packard CJ, Shepherd J. The hepatobiliary axis and lipoprotein metabolism: effects of bile acid sequestrants and ileal by-pass surgery. *J Lipid Res* 1982;23:1081–1098.

11. Witztum JL, Schonfeld G, Weidman SW. The effects of colestipol on the metabolism of very low density lipoproteins in man. *J Lab Clin Med* 1976;88:1008–1018.
12. Angelin B, Leijd B, Hultcrantz R, Einarsson K. Increased turnover of very low density lipoprotein triglyceride during treatment with cholestyramine in familial hypercholesterolaemia. *J Intern Med* 1990;227:201–206.
13. Illingworth DR, Bacon SP, Larsen KK. Long-term experience with HMG-CoA reductase inhibitors in the therapy of hypercholesterolemia. *Atheroscler Rev* 1988;18:161–187.
14. Rudling M, Reihnér E, Einarsson K, Ewerth S, Angelin B. Low density lipoprotein receptor binding activity in human tissues: quantitative importance of hepatic receptors and evidence for regulation of their expression in vivo. *Proc Natl Acad Sci USA* 1990;87:3469–3473.
15. Angelin B, Björkhem I, Einarsson K. Influence of bile acids on the soluble phosphatidic acid phosphatase in rat liver. *Biochem Biophys Res Commun* 1981;180:606–612.
16. Melish J, Le N-A, Ginsberg H, Steinberg D, Brown MV. Dissociation of apoprotein B and triglyceride production in very low density lipoproteins. *Am J Physiol* 1980;239:E354–62.
17. Grundy SM, Mok HYI, Zech L, Steinberg D, Berman M. Transport of very low density lipoprotein triglycerides in varying degrees of obesity and hypertriglyceridemia. *J Clin Invest* 1979;63:1274–1283.
18. Angelin B, Hershon KC, Brunzell JD. Bile acid metabolism in hereditary forms of hypertriglyceridemia: evidence for an increased synthesis rate in monogenic familial hypertriglyceridemia. *Proc Natl Acad Sci USA* 1987;44:5434–5438.
19. Vega GL, Grundy SM. Studies on mechanisms for enhanced clearance of low density lipoproteins in patients with primary hypertriglyceridemia. *J Intern Med* 1989;226:5–15.
20. Kekki M. Plasma triglyceride turnover in 92 adult normolipidaemic and 30 hypertriglyceridemic subjects—the effect of age, synthesis rate and removal capacity on plasma triglyceride concentration. *Ann Clin Res* 1980;12:64–76.

Atherosclerosis Reviews, Volume 22,
edited by A. M. Gotto, Jr. and R. Paoletti.
Raven Press, Ltd., New York © 1991.

Biguanides in Hypertriglyceridemia and in the Management of Arterial Disease

Cesare R. Sirtori and Maria Rosa Lovati

Center E. Grossi Paoletti, Institute of Pharmacological Sciences, University of Milano, 20133 Milano, Italy

Biguanides are guanidine derivatives that have been in clinical use for the treatment of type II diabetes for the past 30 years. Of the three molecules developed for this indication—phenformin, metformin, and buformin—only the first two are currently available in the clinic. Phenformin is used mostly in fixed-dose combination therapies with a sulfonylurea in a few countries; by contrast, metformin is widely used as monotherapy or in combination therapy in many European and American nations.

The effect of biguanides on glycemic regulation differs from that of sulfonylureas. Whereas sulfonylureas act mainly by stimulating the insulin secretion of pancreatic β-cells (1), biguanides act primarily by peripheral mechanisms. Although an effect on intestinal glucose absorption has by now been excluded with certainty (2), the drug's action on the peripheral metabolism of glucose seems more significant. Biguanides act by inhibiting gluconeogenesis, stimulating tissue glucose uptake as well as anaerobic glycolysis (3,4). An increase in the number of peripheral insulin receptors after metformin treatment has also been reported (5). However, the effect on insulin-stimulated glucose utilization occurs in an identical way in patients with type I and type II diabetes (6), thus suggesting that the drug acts directly (7).

With metformin, the increase of lactic acid levels, a consequence of the enhanced anaerobic glycolysis, is generally of a minor degree and transient (8). In the case of phenformin, lactacidemia may, at times, be significant and even life-threatening (9). This effect is due to the presence in the population of 8% to 10% of individuals with a reduced capacity to parahydroxylate phenformin, in order to facilitate renal disposal (10). Poor metabolizers of phenformin run an enhanced risk of lactic acidosis that can prove fatal. Because of this danger, phenformin has been withdrawn from clinical use in most Western countries. In contrast, metformin, which does not undergo liver metabolism, but only renal clearance (filtration + tubular secretion) (11), has rarely been associated with lactic acidosis; not a single case has been reported in Canada for the past 20 years (12).

Detailed clinical studies and a chance experimental observation have paved the way for new indications for the use of metformin. The major use is in hypertriglyceridemia; the second, stemming both from experimental data on cholesterol-fed rabbits and also from clinical observations in patients, is in the management of peripheral arterial disease. The effect of the drug on lipid status and vascular parameters may be related.

METFORMIN IN HYPERTRIGLYCERIDEMIA

The very early studies on phenformin in obesity and diabetes indicated that this drug might, in some cases, improve plasma lipid status (13). A controlled study carried out by Gustafson et al. (14) suggested instead that metformin (1.5 g daily for a minimal duration of 4 months) could significantly reduce triglyceridemia in both type IV and type IIB patients. This decrease (around 26%) was accompanied by a reduction in basal plasma insulin levels, as well as in the sum of plasma insulin levels after an oral glucose tolerance test (OGTT). No significant changes were noted in fasting blood glucose; indeed, there was even an increase in the sum of glucose levels during OGTT in type IIB patients. The authors noted that the plasma lipid reduction was not associated with a significant reduction in body weight. This study, whose major flaw was the relatively low triglyceride (TG) levels in the treated patients, was followed by an extensive investigation by Fedele et al. (15) in type IV patients with more consistent hypertriglyceridemia. In these cases, after 3 months of treatment, the TG reduction averaged about 40%. Interestingly, also in this study, there were minimal changes in plasma glucose levels, and plasma insulin was significantly reduced only in patients with fasting hyperglycemia, not those with chemical diabetes.

In an effort to describe the clinical profile of patients most likely to respond to the hypoglyceridemic effect of metformin, Sirtori et al. (16), in a series of 30 patients with stable hypertriglyceridemia (types IIB and IV) and variable degrees of glucose intolerance, identified 18 subjects with a hypotriglyceridemic effect exceeding 30% ("responders") and 12 where the effect was negligible ("nonresponders") (Fig. 1). The nonresponders had a higher body weight and plasma cholesterol (Fig. 2) and, showed a glycemic response to OGTT of a diabetic type (Fig. 3). In both responders and nonresponders, the sum of insulin values after glucose was significantly reduced. This study indicated that the TG-lowering effect of metformin was likely to be related to a decreased lipoprotein secretion, with a limited correlation with the reduced insulinemia.

The positive effect of metformin on triglyceridemia was later confirmed by Descovich et al. (17) in a series of 260 patients with hyperlipoproteinemias types IIA, IIB, and IV. In all hyperlipoproteinemia phenotypes, metformin significantly reduced triglyceridemia, with a minimal effect on plasma cho-

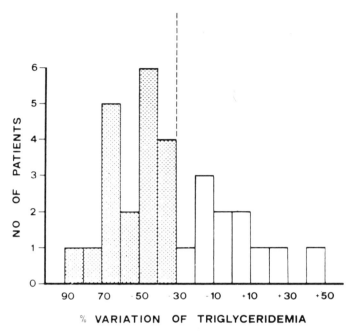

FIG. 1. Distribution of responders (dotted columns) and nonresponders (open columns) among 30 hypertriglyceridemic patients treated with metformin (850 mg t.i.d.) (16).

lesterol. In this, as well as in the prior study, no significant changes were recorded in the low-density lipoprotein (LDL) cholesterol levels of treated patients, thus ruling out a fibric acid–like effect on lipoprotein lipase (18). As a follow-up of the large study (17), Montaguti et al. (19) investigated ECG changes after a longer-term use of the drug. There was a clear reduction in ECG signs of myocardial ischemia in over one-half of the treated patients.

The mechanism of the TG reduction by metformin does not appear to be closely linked to an improved glycemic control in these otherwise mostly normoglycemic patients. TG reduction therefore can probably be explained by a primary effect of the drug on lipoprotein secretion, as well as by an improved peripheral effect of insulin. In both studies where triglyceridemia and insulin levels (both basal and post-glucose) were monitored, a clear effect of the drug was noted (15,16). Since metformin has been shown to increase insulin receptor binding both *in vitro* and *in vivo* (5), as well as to enhance the insulin action *in vivo* (7), it can be expected that it would reduce the insulin resistance and hyperinsulinemia characteristic of type IV patients (20).

To verify this mechanism in an experimental model, Zavaroni et al. (21) tested the effect of metformin on the hypertriglyceridemia induced by fruc-

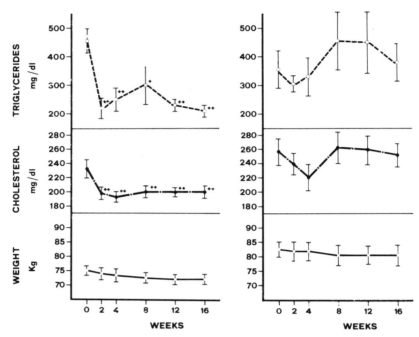

FIG. 2. Sex, age, plasma lipids, and body weight of the (**left**) 18 responders (male, aged 44.8 ± 1.7 years) to metformin and of the (**right**) 12 nonresponders (11 male, 1 female, aged 47.7 ± 2.7 years) (16). A transient lipid-lowering action of the drug is noted in nonresponders who otherwise only show a higher body weight than the responders.

tose in rats. In this condition, both hyperinsulinemia and insulin resistance are found (22). Metformin fully prevented both the insulin and TG rises induced by the experimental diet. By monitoring the very-low-density lipoprotein (VLDL)-TG secretion rate, a preventive effect on the hypersecretion induced by the dietary saccharide could be shown. We can thus conclude that metformin most likely reduces plasma TG by lowering basal or stimulated insulin levels and/or increasing the peripheral insulin activity, in this way regulating VLDL hypersecretion. By this mechanism, the effect of the drug is not necessarily restricted to diabetic individuals, but may be found in all patient groups.

An additional observation of interest relates to the apolipoprotein changes induced by metformin in patients. In a parallel evaluation of VLDL composition in cholesterol-fed rabbits (see below) and patients with type III hyperlipoproteinemia (who have a VLDL composition similar to the experimental model), metformin remarkably reduced VLDL apolipoprotein E (VLDL-apoE) in both (23). The striking reduction of VLDL-apoE in type III patients thus suggests, as is also demonstrated in the rabbit model, that intestinal lipoprotein secretion may be modified by the treatment (24).

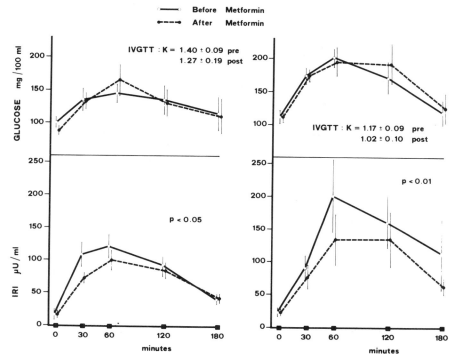

FIG. 3. Means ± SEM of glucose and insulin levels of metformin responders (**left**) and nonresponders (**right**) following OGTT (16). Nonresponders clearly show a diabetic OGTT; whereas in both cases, metformin significantly reduces the sum of insulin values after glucose without altering the K coefficient.

METFORMIN IN PERIPHERAL VASCULAR DISEASE

Two chance observations helped to establish this potential use of metformin in clinical disease. First, Agid and Marquié reported that metformin could exert a surprising protective effect on atheromatosis development in cholesterol-fed rabbits (25). This observation, supported by a variety of basic studies by our group, provided the stimulus to further evaluate the drug in clinical conditions. Apparently, the prevention of cholesterol atheromatosis in rabbits is related to dramatic changes in VLDL composition. VLDL become less enriched with cholesteryl esters and with apoE (i.e., in a similar fashion to the above-described clinical observation in type III) (26). VLDL from cholesterol-metformin–treated rabbits have an increased catabolism and a reduced uptake by the arterial wall (27).

When examining hypertriglyceridemic patients with peripheral vascular disease, it soon became obvious that many of them reported a dramatic

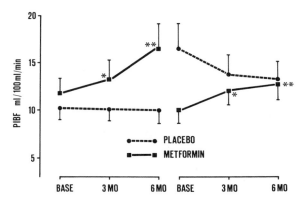

FIG. 4. Changes of postischemic blood fow (PIBF) to the extremities (22 limbs, X̄ ± SEM) before and after metformin (850 t.i.d.) or placebo in 15 patients with peripheral arterial disease participating in a cross-over trial with the drug (28); *$p < 0.05$; **$p < 0.001$ versus respective baselines.

improvement of their conditions, which were stable over a prolonged period of time. These anecdotal observations, confirmed within the large clinical trial with the drug (17), were later the object of a controlled clinical study. In this study (28), the activity of metformin was tested in a group of patients with established peripheral vascular disease who were monitored by quantitative strain-gauge plethysmography, an objective method evaluating total flow to the extremities before and after different treatments. This cross-over trial (two periods of 6 months of drug or placebo treatment, separated by a 1 month washout), clearly indicated that metformin administration was associated with a 20% to 30% improvement of the peak postischemic blood flow to the affected extremities (Fig. 4). Changes of triglyceridemia were minimal; patients generally had TG levels in the normal range. However, an interesting high-density lipoprotein (HDL) rise (9% as the mean of the two sequences) was noted; this was accompanied by a rise in the apoA-I-1 isoprotein in isoelectric focusing gels of separated HDL (28).

In addition to the lipid/insulin changes following drug treatment, another potential therapeutic mechanism of metformin is by way of activation of fibrinolysis. Fibrinolytic activity is typically reduced in type IV patients because of increased levels of plasminogen activator inhibitor type 1 (PAI-1), the major inhibitor of fibrinolysis (29). Studies with metformin in obese hypertriglyceridemic patients have shown a characteristic reduction of the inhibitor after treatment (30). In an ongoing study in patients with arterial disease, who were treated with a very low dose of metformin (500 mg b.i.d.), we found an improved vascular function in the extremities, as well as a consistent, sustained reduction of PAI-1.

Metformin may provide an exciting tool for the physiological evaluation and for treatment of vascular disease. Numerous contributions, which have been collected in a monograph (31), show that metformin can improve spontaneous vasomotion when it is altered by different stimuli (hypoxia, anesthesia, etc.) (32). Even with very low concentrations of the drug, researchers report improved vascular mobility and the repair of lesions induced by experimental diabetes, ischemia, or other pathological conditions in the experimental animal. The therapeutic potential of this old drug, which costs very little and has a relatively wide range of indications, is probably largely unexplored.

REFERENCES

1. Gierich JE. Oral hypoglycemic agents. *N Engl J Med* 1989;321:1231–1245.
2. Olsen WA, Rasmussen HK. Effect of phenformin on carbohydrate absorption in man. *Diabetes* 1974;23:716–718.
3. Hermann LS. Metformin: a review of its pharmacological properties and therapeutic use. *Diab Metab* 1979;3:233–245.
4. Prager R, Schernthaner G, Graf H. Effect of metformin on peripheral glucose utilization in noninsulin-dependent diabetes mellitus. *Metabolism* 1987;36:774–776.
5. Holle AW, Mangels M, Dreyer J, Kuhnau HW, Rudinger HW. Biguanide treatment increases the number of insulin-receptor sites on human erythrocytes. *N Engl J Med* 1981;305:563–566.
6. Gin H, Messerschmitt C, Brottier E, Aubertin J. Metformin improved insulin resistance in type I, insulin-dependent, diabetic patients. *Metabolism* 1985;10:923–925.
7. Hother-Nielsen O, Schmitz O, Andersen PH, Beck-Nielsen H, Pedersen O. Metformin improves peripheral, but not hepatic insulin action in obese patients with type II diabetes. *Acta Endocrinol* 1989;120:257–265.
8. Luft D, Schmülling RM, Eggstein M. Lactic acidosis in biguanide-treated diabetes. *Diabetologia* 1978;14:75–87.
9. Alberti KGMM, Nattrass M. Lactic acidosis. *Lancet* 1977;2:25–29.
10. Bosisio E, Galli-Kienle M, Galli G, et al. Defective hydroxylation of phenformin as a determinant of drug toxicity. *Diabetes* 1981;30:644–649.
11. Sirtori CR, Franceschini G, Galli-Kienle M, Galli G, Bondioli A, Conti F. Disposition of metformin (N, N-dimethylbiguanide) in man. *Clin Pharmacol Ther* 1978;24:683–693.
12. Vigneri R, Goldfine ID. Role of metformin in treatment of diabetes mellitus. *Diabetes Care* 1987;10:118–122.
13. Tzagournis M, Chiles R, Ryan JM, Skillmann TG. Interrelationships of hyperinsulinism and hypertriglyceridemia in young patients with coronary artery disease. *Circulation* 1968;38:1156–1163.
14. Gustafson A, Björntorp P, Falhen M. Metformin administration in hyperlipidemic states. *Acta Med Scand* 1971;190:491–494.
15. Fedele S, Tiengo A, Nosadini R, et al. Hypolipidemic effects of metformin in hyperprebetalipoproteinemia. *Diab Metab* 1976;2:127–134.
16. Sirtori CR, Tremoli E, Sirtori M, Conti F, Paoletti R. Treatment of hypertriglyceridemia with metformin. Effectiveness and analysis of results. *Atherosclerosis* 1977;26:583–592.
17. Descovich GC, Montaguti U, Ceredi C, Cocuzza E, Sirtori CR. Long-term treatment with metformin in a large cohort of hyperlipidemic patients. *Artery* 1978;4:348–359.
18. Sirtori CR, Franceschini G. Effects of fibrates on serum lipids and atherosclerosis. *Pharmacol Ther* 1988;37:167–191.
19. Montaguti U, Celin D, Ceredi C, Descovich GC. Efficacy of the long-term administration of metformin in hyperlipidaemic patients. *Res Clin Forums* 1979;1:95–103.
20. Olefsky JM, Farquhar GM, Reaven GM. Reappraisal of the role of insulin in hypertriglyceridemia. *Am J Med* 1974;57:551–560.
21. Zavaroni I, Dall'Aglio E, Bruschi F, Alpi O, Coscelli C, Butturini U. Inhibition of carbohydrate-induced hypertriglyceridemia by metformin. *Horm Metab Res* 1984;16:85–87.
22. Zavaroni I, Sander S, Scott S, Reaven GM. Effect of fructose feeding on insulin secretion and insulin action in the rat. *Metabolism* 1980;29:970–973.
23. Sirtori CR, Catapano, Ghiselli GC, Shore B, Shore VG. Effects of metformin on lipoprotein composition in rabbits and man. *Prot Biol Fluids* 1978;25:379–383.

24. Weber G, Catapano A, Ghiselli GC, Sirtori CR. Experimental studies on the antiatheros- clerotic effect of metformin. In: Carlson LA, Paoletti, R, Sictori CR, Weber Y, eds. *International conference on atherosclerosis*. New York: Raven, 1978;319–325.
25. Agid R, Marquié G. Effects préventifs du NN-diméthyl-biguanide sur le développement de l'athérosclérose induite par le cholestérol chez le lapin. *C R Acad Sci* (III) 1969;269:1000– 1011.
26. Sirtori CR, Catapano A, Ghiselli GC, Innocenti AL, Rodriguez J. Metformin: an antiath- erosclerotic agent modifying very low density lipoproteins in rabbits. *Atherosclerosis* 1977;26:79–89.
27. Rodriguez J, Catapano A, Ghiselli GC, Sirtori CR. Turnover and aortic uptake of very low density lipoproteins (VLDL) from hypercholesterolemic rabbits as a model for testing an- tiatherosclerotic compounds. *Adv Exp Med Biol* 1976;67:169–189.
28. Sirtori CR, Franceschini G, Gianfranceschi G, et al. Metformin improves peripheral vas- cular flow in non hyperlipidemic patients with arterial disease. *J Cardiovasc Pharmacol* 1984;6:914–923.
29. Sundell IB, Nilsson TK, Hallmans G, Hellsten G, Dahlen G. Interrelationships between plasma levels of plasminogen activator inhibitor, lipoprotein (a), and established cardio- vascular risk factors in a North Swedish population. *Atherosclerosis* 1989;80:9–16.
30. Vague P, Juhar-Vague I, Alessi MC, Badier C, Valadier J. Metformin decreases the elevated levels of plasminogen activator inhibitor, plasma insulin and triglyceride in non diabetic obese subjects. *Thromb Haemost* 1987;57:326–328.
31. Intaglietta M. Sirtori CR, Standl E, Vague P. Vascular disease and diabetes mellitus. A new approach. *Diab Metab* 1988;14(suppl 4).
32. Intaglietta M. Arteriolar vasomotion: normal physiological activity or defense? *Diab Metab* 1988;14:489–494.

Atherosclerosis Reviews, Volume 22,
edited by A. M. Gotto, Jr. and R. Paoletti.
Raven Press, Ltd., New York © 1991.

The Influence of Fibrates on Lipoprotein Metabolism

James Shepherd, Bruce Griffin, Muriel Caslake, Allan Gaw, and Christopher Packard

Institute of Biochemistry, Royal Infirmary, Glasgow G4 OSF, Scotland

Clofibrate was launched as a lipid-lowering agent over 30 years ago. Its success provided an important stimulus for the development of a series of second- and third-generation analogues (Fig. 1) that have captured a substantial proportion of the market worldwide. Although they all share the primary actions of their progenitor in lowering plasma triglyceride (TG) and cholesterol, they have varying hypolipidemic potencies and different influences on such diverse phenomena as bile lithogenicity (1,2), plasma fibrinogen (3), and glycemic control (4). Undoubtedly, these differences depend in part on substantial variations in the pharmacokinetics of drug handling (Fig. 2); nevertheless, it is clear that each fibrate offers unique benefits and actions, depending on the clinical circumstances. As a group, however, they exert a limited number of primary effects on all major lipoprotein species in the circulation. By promoting the lipolysis of TG-rich particles (5) and limiting the availability of free fatty acids (FFA) for the synthesis of TG in the liver (6), they exert their principal action—the lowering of plasma TG.

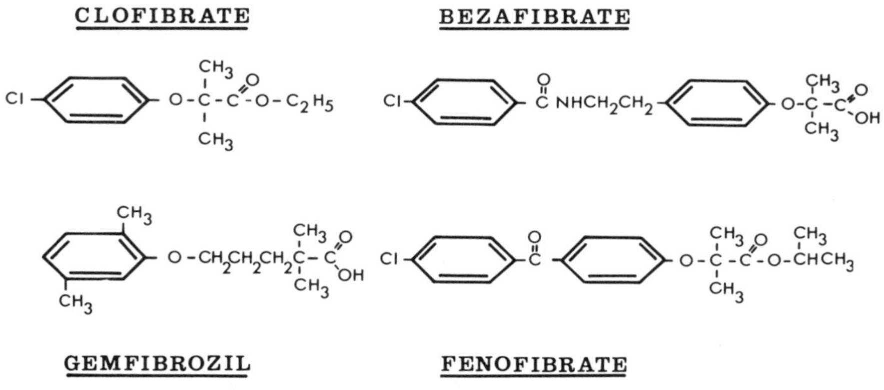

FIG. 1. Structural formulae of the commonly used fibrates.

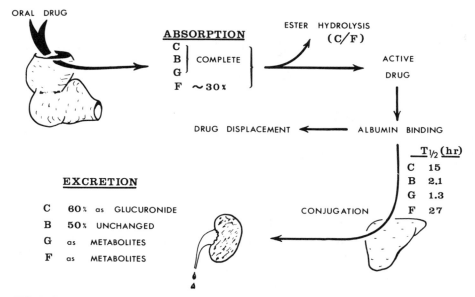

FIG. 2. Pharmacokinetics of the fibrates. Key: C = clofibrate; B = bezafibrate; G = gemfibrozil; F = fenofibrate.

In addition, they may be responsible for indirect suppression of the synthesis of cholesterol in the liver (7). These effects give rise to a series of secondary responses in lipoprotein metabolism that require further elucidation (Fig. 3).

FIBRATES IN CLINICAL PRACTICE

It is not surprising that, in the past, concern has been expressed over the common finding that plasma low-density lipoprotein (LDL) cholesterol, a widely accepted index of coronary heart disease (CHD) risk, often rises when fibrates are given to hypertriglyceridemic patients. However, recent studies have revealed that LDL is both structurally and metabolically heterogeneous. In the plasma of all normal and hyperlipidemic individuals, LDL exists as a group of distinct subfractions (8,9) that can be distinguished on the basis of particle size and density, as LDL_1, LDL_2, and LDL_3. A preponderance of small, dense LDL (LDL_3), in combination with raised TG, has been linked to an increased predisposition to myocardial infarction (MI) (10). Therefore, the CHD risk associated with raised LDL levels cannot be fully assessed without detailed examination and knowledge of the metabolism and structure of these LDL subfractions.

As our clinical experience of the fibrates develops, we have come to expect differing responses to their use depending on the type and degree of

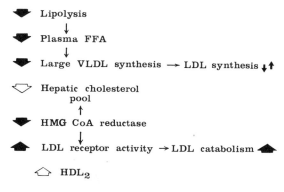

FIG. 3. Effects of clofibrate analogues on lipoprotein metabolism. A variety of actions have been ascribed to the clofibrate analogues. By inhibiting adipose tissue lipolysis, they reduce the flux of free fatty acids to the liver and limit substrate availability for VLDL synthesis. Hepatic cholesterol metabolism is also affected, leading to activation of LDL receptors and a consequent increase in the rate of catabolism of the lipoprotein. A satisfactory explanation for the increment in HDL that accompanies treatment has not yet been forthcoming.

lipid abnormality under treatment. In this context, it is useful to review independently their differential effects on hypertriglyceridemia and hypercholesterolemia.

FIBRATE THERAPY FOR HYPERTRIGLYCERIDEMIA

The high plasma TG levels characteristically seen in type IV and type V hyperlipoproteinemic subjects result from an increase in the number of large, TG-rich particles in their circulation. Although levels of LDL cholesterol and apolipoprotein B (apoB) are usually normal or even subnormal, structural studies have shown that these particles are unusually small and dense (11). There is evidence to suggest that the principal underlying metabolic lesion in this situation is an overproduction of very-low-density lipoprotein (VLDL) in the liver, accompanied by hypercatabolism of LDL (Table 1). The high rate of LDL clearance is believed to occur through non–receptor-mediated and potentially atherogenic pathways (12).

Treatment with bezafibrate (13) effectively corrects the hypertriglyceridemia by stimulating lipoprotein lipase to promote the removal of VLDL

TABLE 1. *Effects of bezafibrate on apoB kinetics in subjects with hypertriglyceridemia*

	VLDL		IDL		LDL	
	Pool size mg/dl	FCR pools/d	Pool size mg/dl	FCR pools/d	Pool size mg/dl	FCR pools/d
Control	10.5 ± 10.8	7.0 ± 7.5	30.0 ± 6.2	1.23 ± 0.55	55 ± 28	0.47 ± 0.25
Bezafibrate	3.1 ± 3.6	22.9 ± 24.0	38.9 ± 11.5	0.98 ± 0.38	76 ± 22	0.35 ± 0.12
	$p < 0.05$	$p < 0.05$	$p < 0.05$	NS	NS	$p < 0.005$

$n = 6$.

TABLE 2. *Fibrates and hypertriglyceridemia: effects on VLDL*

	Trigylceride[a] mmol/L	Triglyceride/apoB ratio	Particle size
Control	18.3 ± 16.7	34.9 ± 23.5	
Drug	4.8 ± 3.5	9.5 ± 4.2	↓
Change	74% ↓	73% ↓	

n = 6.

triglyceride (Table 1). In so doing, the rate of conversion of VLDL to intermediate-density lipoprotein (IDL) is increased. VLDL synthesis, however, remains unchanged. As far as LDL is concerned, bezafibrate induces an increase in its circulating mass by suppressing its high rate of clearance rather than by influencing its formation from TG-rich precursors (VLDL and IDL).

Fenofibrate therapy (12) produces similar results to those achieved by bezafibrate, establishing a principal and common function for these two agents in facilitating the lipolysis of VLDL TG. Both drugs suppress the hypercatabolism of LDL via non–receptor-mediated pathways while at the same time activating clearance of LDL by receptors. The outcome—normalization of initially low levels of plasma LDL—is accompanied by a significant alteration in LDL composition. The particles become enriched in cholesterol ester and relatively depleted in phospholipid and TG, thereby increasing the lipid core/coat ratio. This change in lipid composition is consistent with an increase in LDL particle size, away from the small, dense LDL characteristic of hypertriglyceridemia (Tables 2 and 3).

HYPERCHOLESTEROLEMIA; THE EFFECTS OF FENOFIBRATE

In normotriglyceridemic individuals with raised blood cholesterol levels, plasma TG is unremarkable whereas LDL cholesterol and apoB are elevated. Kinetic analysis has attributed these raised levels of LDL to a reduced rate of catabolism. Despite these high levels, LDL composition and subfraction distribution is normal.

Treatment of these subjects with fenofibrate consistently lowers plasma

TABLE 3. *Fibrates and hypertriglyceridemia: effects on LDL*

	Cholesterol mmol/L	Cholesterol/apoB ratio	Particle size
Control	1.92 ± 0.91	0.96 ± 0.37	
Drug	2.70 ± 0.70	1.17 ± 0.17	↑
Change	41% ↑	22% ↑	

n = 7.

TG, LDL cholesterol, and apoB. In this case, the fibrate enhances the fractional catabolic rate of LDL by both the receptor- and non–receptor-mediated pathways. In contrast to its effect in hypertriglyceridemia, fenofibrate has no influence on LDL composition. However, analysis of LDL subfractions by high resolution density gradient centrifugation and gradient gel electrophoresis reveals a significant redistribution of LDL density and size toward lighter and larger particles.

The total mass of LDL is reduced as a result of a significant decrease in the LDL subfraction of mid density and size (LDL$_2$). The change in the LDL subfractions of lower density (LDL$_1$) and higher density (LDL$_3$) are inversely related, the most consistent finding being an increase in LDL$_1$ and a decrease in LDL$_3$.

CONCLUSIONS

The putative actions of the fibrates on apoB metabolism are summarized in Fig. 4. Both bezafibrate and fenofibrate significantly lower plasma TG by promoting the lipolysis of TG-rich lipoproteins and increasing the rate of

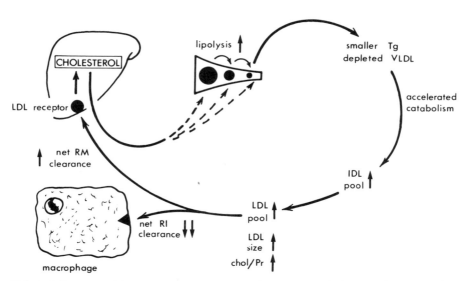

FIG. 4. Influence of fibrates on the metabolism of apolipoprotein B–containing particles in hypertriglyceridemia. Hypertriglyceridemia results from a combination of overproduction and defective catabolism of triglyceride–rich VLDL particles. This leads to reductions in the circulating mass of IDL and LDL, with concomitant structural compositional changes in the latter. Fibrates reverse these defects, accelerating VLDL lipolysis and promoting its conversion to IDL and LDL. This restores to normality the composition and size of the LDL particles in the circulation. RM: receptor mediated; RI: receptor independent.

conversion of VLDL to IDL. In severe hypertriglyceridemia, the fibrates induce an increase in LDL cholesterol and apoB by suppressing its hyper-catabolism via non–receptor-mediated pathways. This results in a restoration of plasma LDL cholesterol and the overall composition of LDL toward normal as well as an activation of the net clearance of LDL by receptors. In contrast, in hypercholesterolemia, fenofibrate corrects the high levels of LDL by stimulating its fractional catabolic rate.

In both hyperlipemic states, the fibrates redistribute LDL density and size toward lighter and larger particles. When these structural changes are interpreted as quantative differences in defined LDL subfractions, fenofibrate induces an LDL profile that has been associated with a lower coronary risk.

The clinical efficacy of the fibrate gemfibrozil has been successfully demonstrated in the Helsinki Heart Study (14). We can predict from the effects of bezafibrate and fenofibrate on lipoprotein metabolism that these hypolipidemic agents should be at least as effective in influencing coronary morbidity.

ACKNOWLEDGMENTS

We thank Claire McKerron for her expert secretarial help. This work was supported by grants from the British Heart Foundation (87/101, 87/6, 89/107) and the Scottish Hospital Endowments Research Trust (908).

REFERENCES

1. Hunninghake DB, Peters JR. Effect of fibric acid derivatives on blood lipids and lipoprotein levels. *Am J Med* 1987;83(suppl 5B):44–49.
2. Palmer RH. Effects of fibric acid derivatives on biliary lipid composition. *Am J Med* 1987;83(suppl 5B):37–43.
3. Almer LO, Kjellstrom T. The fibrinolytic system and coagulation during bezafibrate treatment of hypertriglyceridemia. *Atherosclerosis* 1986;61:81–85.
4. Study Group of the European Atherosclerosis Society. The recognition and management of hyperlipidaemia in adults; a policy statement of the EAS. *Eur Heart J* 1988;9:571–600.
5. Wolfe BM, Kane JP, Havel RJ, Brewster HP. Mechanism of the hyperlipidemic effect of clofibrate in postabsorptive man. *J Clin Invest* 1973;52:2146–2159.
6. Rifkind BM. Effect of CPIB ester on plasma free fatty acid levels in man. *Metabolism* 1966;15:673–675.
7. Bernt J, Gaumert R, Still J. Mode of action of the lipid lowering agents clofibrate and BM 15.075 on cholesterol biosynthesis in rat liver. *Atherosclerosis* 1978;30:147–152.
8. Krauss RM, Burke DJ. Identification of multiple subclasses of plasma lipoproteins in normal humans. *J Lipid Res* 1981;23:97–104.
9. Fisher WR. Heterogeneity of plasma low density lipoproteins. Manifestations of the physiological phenomenon in man. *Metabolism* 1983;32:283–291.
10. Austin MA, Breslow JL, Hennekens CH. Low density lipoprotein subclass patterns and risk of myocardial infarction. *JAMA* 1988;260:1917–1921.
11. Eisenberg S, Gavish D, Oschry Y, Fainaru M, Deckelbaum RJ. Abnormalities in very low, low and high density lipoproteins in hypertriglyceridemia. Reversal towards normal with bezafibrate treatment. *J Clin Invest* 1984;74:470–479.

12. Shepherd J, Caslake MJ, Lorimer AR, Vallance BD, Packard CJ. Fenofibrate reduces low density lipoprotein catabolism in hypertriglyceridemic subjects. *Arteriosclerosis* 1985;5:162–168.
13. Shepherd J, Packard CJ, Stewart JM, et al. Apolipoprotein A and B (Sf 100–400) metabolism during bezafibrate therapy in hypertriglyceridemic subjects. *J Clin Invest* 1984;74:2164–2177.

Atherosclerosis Reviews, Volume 22,
edited by A. M. Gotto, Jr. and R. Paoletti.
Raven Press, Ltd., New York © 1991.

Treatment of Hypertriglyceridemia

Exercise

Peter D. Wood

*Stanford Center for Research in Disease Prevention, Stanford University,
Stanford, California 94305*

A considerable body of research, especially that of Morris, in England (1), and Paffenbarger, in the United States (2), indicates that adult men who engage in regular, moderate exercise have a considerably reduced risk of fatal heart attack. The Lipid Research Clinics Follow-Up Study (3) and, recently, Blair et al. (4) have shown that level of physical fitness in both men and women (measured by treadmill testing) has a strong negative correlation with coronary heart disease (CHD). Rate of total mortality is considerably greater in the less fit (and especially in the least fit) compared with the more fit. Thus, it appears that even modest increases in exercise and fitness level among our most sedentary citizens yield substantial health dividends.

In discussing exercise, we should remember that the regular exerciser exhibits other characteristics that are difficult to disentangle from increased muscular contraction per se (5)—i.e., leanness and a relatively high caloric intake per kilogram of body weight. This overview of the role of exercise in hypertriglyceridemia does not review work done to separate exercise from changes in body composition because, from a practical point of view, the exhortation to "take exercise and lose weight" is a single prescription. Also, it is difficult to imagine an exercise training study of any length in which not only body weight but also total body fat and the distribution of that fat are unchanged relative to control.

EXERCISE, PLASMA TRIGLYCERIDES, AND CHD RISK

The evidence is quite persuasive that the salutary effect of regular exercise on CHD risk is due in part to changes in the concentrations of lipoprotein classes in the blood. Exercise (with accompanying loss of body fat) results in many changes in lipoprotein concentrations, including those of total plasma triglycerides (TG) and of the TG-rich very-low-density lipoproteins

(VLDL). It should also be remembered that total volume of plasma increases significantly with increased exercise level—a fact that must be taken into account when changes in the total plasma content of a given lipoprotein are under consideration.

In the Framingham Study, risk of CHD increases for men and women on 30-year follow-up across the concentration range from normal to moderately elevated TG—i.e., from approximately 1.4 to 3.4 mmol/L or 120 to 300 mg/dl. The independence (or otherwise) of this association has been a much-discussed topic. Obesity and concomitant sedentary living are generally regarded as the major causes of moderate TG elevation, which is very common in developed countries. Although attainment of a healthy body weight through diet and exercise is a primary goal in treatment of hypertriglyceridemia due to secondary causes and genetic hyperlipidemias (6), the greatest gain in public health will probably come from increasing exercise among the very large proportion of individuals who are quite sedentary and moderately hypertriglyceridemic. It is this large group, who are normally not candidates for drug treatment, that will be discussed here.

EXERCISE AND TRIGLYCERIDES: CROSS-SECTIONAL STUDIES

Many comparisons of active versus sedentary people have shown generally lower fasting plasma TG levels in the exercisers. Early studies showed generally low TG level in male and female runners compared to sedentary controls (7), and also demonstrated the generally lower plasma TG in women versus men (8). Exercisers also show substantially higher levels of high-density lipoproteins (HDL), which are inversely related to TG concentrations and predict lower CHD risk, for the active groups (9). The percentage of body fat in exercisers is lower than that for sedentary groups.

During a prevalence study of several thousand staff and faculty on the Stanford University campus, we measured fasting plasma TG and also classified participants by their self-description as "runners," "joggers" or "non-joggers." There was a gradation of TG concentrations from the least active to the most active groups for each sex.

In another cross-sectional comparison (Table 1), in collaboration with Drs. Krauss and Lindgren of the Donner Laboratory, University of California, fasting plasma from 12 male runners and 20 sedentary, age-matched controls was examined for lipoprotein mass distribution by analytical ultracentrifugation. The TG-rich fraction of S_f 20 to 400 (VLDL) was substantially and significantly lower in mass concentration in the runners versus the controls. S_f 0 to 7, the "small" fraction of the low-density lipoproteins (LDL), was also significantly lower in the runners. From these and many other such cross-sectional studies involving walkers, soccer players, swimmers, tennis players, and other active groups, the picture emerges of active people as

TABLE 1. Comparison of age, body mass index, lipids, lipoproteins, lipoprotein lipase, and hepatic lipase measurements in cross-sectional samples of long-distance runners and sedentary men

	Runners (M ± SD)	Nonrunners (M ± SD)	Difference (M ± SE)	Significance (p)
Age (yr)	46.9 ± 7.5	45.7 ± 6.1	1.3 ± 2.3	0.81
Body mass index (kg/m^2)	22.6 ± 2.0	25.1 ± 3.3	−2.5 ± 0.7	0.006
Lipids and lipoproteins				
Plasma total cholesterol (mg/dl)	190.9 ± 36.6	217.0 ± 31.1	−26.1 ± 11.3	0.02
Plasma total triglycerides (mg/dl)	70.8 ± 35.0	123.0 ± 59.3	−52.2 ± 12.5	0.001
Plasma HDL cholesterol (mg/dl)	64.9 ± 12.5	49.6 ± 8.7	15.3 ± 3.8	0.0001
Serum HDL mass of $F_{1.20}$ 0−1.5 (mg/dl)	70.0 ± 13.7	82.3 ± 17.5	−12.3 ± 4.5	0.02
Serum HDL mass of $F_{1.20}$ 1.5−2.0 (mg/dl)	51.2 ± 8.4	52.3 ± 7.8	−1.1 ± 2.6	0.98
Serum HDL mass of $F_{1.20}$ 2.0−9.0 (mg/dl)	213.0 ± 45.6	144.8 ± 47.9	68.2 ± 14.5	0.0002
Plasma LDL cholesterol (mg/dl)	147.0 ± 27.5	161.1 ± 30.7	−30.9 ± 9.5	0.004
Serum LDL mass of S_f 0−7 (mg/dl)	138.4 ± 45.3	227.6 ± 67.9	−89.2 ± 15.6	0.0001
Serum LDL mass of S_f 7−12 (mg/dl)	136.7 ± 39.8	134.2 ± 43.8	2.5 ± 12.7	0.85
Serum IDL mass of S_f 12−20 (mg/dl)	34.3 ± 18.2	43.8 ± 20.7	−9.5 ± 5.9	0.16
Plasma VLDL cholesterol (mg/dl)	9.1 ± 8.3	20.4 ± 11.7	−11.3 ± 2.8	0.001
Serum VLDL mass of S_f 20−400 (mg/dl)	36.8 ± 41.6	106.1 ± 72.0	−69.3 ± 15.0	0.001
Postheparin lipase activity				
Lipoprotein lipase (mEq fatty acid/ml/h)	5.0 ± 1.8	3.6 ± 1.2	1.4 ± 0.6	0.04
Hepatic lipase (mEq fatty acid/ml/h)	4.1 ± 2.1	6.5 ± 2.6	−2.4 ± 0.9	0.02

From ref. 13 with permission.
Sample sizes are 12 runners and 64 nonrunners for all lipid and lipoprotein variables, age, and body mass index and 12 runners and 16 nonrunners for lipoprotein and hepatic lipase measurements. All significance levels are obtained from two-sample Wilcoxon sign rank tests.

favored with respect to the atherogenic potential of their plasma lipoprotein mix. In particular, in relation to the topic of this symposium, their VLDL fractions are often remarkably low in concentration compared to sedentary controls.

Plasma concentrations of apolipoprotein A-I (apoA-I), the principal apoprotein of HDL, are generally higher, while apolipoprotein B (apoB) concentrations tend to be lower in lean, active individuals compared to sedentary individuals.

Postheparin lipoprotein lipase generally displays higher activity and hepatic lipase lower activity in lean, active men and women compared to sedentary people (Table 1).

EXERCISE AND TRIGLYCERIDES: TRAINING STUDIES

Many training (intervention) studies have been reported, the majority in adult men, in which the effect of an exercise program on plasma lipoprotein concentrations has been measured. The more persuasive studies, in my view, meet the following minimum criteria: (a) Adequate training period to allow for increase in fitness to a level where a reasonable degree of exercise can be performed regularly. This translates into a study measured in months rather than weeks. (b) Use of a control group, with random assignment to exercise or control. (c) Appropriate statistical analysis of data.

It appears to be impossible to use a double-blind design in such trials. A long-term exercise trial without changes in body composition and caloric intake defies the imagination.

Sound trials generally support the cross-sectional findings and indicate reduction of plasma total TG, VLDL total mass (by analytical ultracentrifugation), and VLDL triglycerides, with increase in HDL total mass and HDL cholesterol with sustained increase in physical activity (9). This is particularly true for individuals who are overweight and who show moderate elevations of plasma TG initially. Individuals who are relatively slim initially and have normal TG levels (< 120 mg/dl) show minimal decreases in TG.

In a recent 1-year trial by our group (10) in moderately overweight men (120–160% of "ideal" weight; aged 30–59 years), 42 were randomly assigned to no-treatment control; 42 to lose significant body fat by caloric restriction without change in quality of diet or exercise level; and 47 to lose significant body fat by progressive exercise without dietary changes. Measurements of body composition, fasting plasma lipids and lipoproteins, and fitness were made at baseline and at 1 year in the weight-steady state. Weight loss averaged about 6 kg, and mean decline in percent body fat was not significantly different for the two weight loss groups. Plasma HDL cholesterol increased significantly by about 5 mg/dl (0.13 mmol/L) in both weight loss groups relative to control. TG levels fell significantly by 31 mg/dl (0.35 mmol/L) in the diet group and by 21 mg/dl (0.24 mmol/L) in the exercise group. We concluded that loss of body fat, whether accomplished by caloric restriction alone or by increased exercise alone results in comparable reductions in plasma TG in men with normal or moderately elevated TG levels.

In a further 1-year study in moderately overweight men and women, as yet unpublished except in abstract form (11), participants were randomly assigned to control (no treatment); to weight loss by caloric restriction on an American Heart Association (AHA) Phase I diet (composed of approximately 55% carbohydrate and 30% fat, emphasizing a major reduction in saturated fat, dietary cholesterol intake of less than 300 mg/day, and adequate fiber intake); or to a diet intervention exactly as described *plus* supervised physical activity including aerobic movement classes, brisk walking, and/or jogging. Men and women in both intervention groups adhered well to the diet, as judged by 7-day food records. The diet plus exercise groups walked and/or ran an average of 15 ± 8.0 km a week and increased their maximum aerobic capacity significantly compared to controls. All intervention groups lost significant body fat compared to controls; in the men, addition of exercise to dietary restriction on the AHA diet produced significantly greater body fat loss than diet alone (− 9.0 kg versus − 5.5 kg, relative to controls). Plasma LDL cholesterol level was reduced in both weight loss groups, relative to controls, although not significantly so for the men. In men, HDL cholesterol was increased relative to controls only in the diet-plus-exercise group. In women, the diet-plus-exercise group showed a significant increase in HDL cholesterol relative to the diet-only group. In men, addition of exercise to diet produced a striking decrease in plasma TG concentration in comparison with diet alone (− 59 versus − 27 mg/dl; − 0.66 versus − 0.30 mmol/L). Our conclusion from this study is that addition of a moderate, progressive exercise component to a long-term dietary weight loss program based on a prudent diet is very useful for overall improvement in plasma lipoprotein status in overweight people with normal to moderately elevated plasma lipoprotein levels. This is particularly true for TG reduction in overweight men.

There is also good evidence that postprandial plasma TG concentrations are substantially reduced in individuals who have lost weight and become fit.

SUMMARY AND PROPOSALS

Adoption by sedentary people of a program of regular aerobic exercise has many salutary effects on lipoprotein metabolism, plasma TG concentration, and other CHD risk factors: (a) There is some evidence that fat distribution is favorably changed by reduction of abdominal obesity, which also is associated with improved plasma lipoprotein pattern (12). (b) Resting and ambulatory blood pressures are frequently decreased. (c) Fasting plasma TG and VLDL total mass are reduced. Postprandial TG levels are reduced by exercise so that arteries are exposed, day in and day out over the decades, to a diminished "tide" of TG-rich particles. (d) LDL cholesterol tends to be low. "Small" LDL of S_f 0 to 7, which appears to be particularly atherogenic, and apoB are lowered. (e) Plasma HDL and HDL_2 cholesterol are increased by exercise and weight loss. ApoA-I is increased. (f) Postheparin lipoprotein lipase activity is increased, and hepatic lipase activity is decreased. (g) Insulin response to a carbohydrate load is reduced, and insulin resistance is much improved by exercise and weight loss.

Exercise could be considered the "all-purpose risk reducer" for CHD. Yet increased physical activity has not been widely used either to reduce risk of CHD or as a way of treating moderate elevations of plasma TG. The U.S. National Cholesterol Education Program's Adult Treatment Guidelines properly emphasize dietary change and (where indicated) drug treatment for elevated cholesterol, but they scarcely mention increasing physical activity. Perhaps this is because there are few commercial sponsors for exercise.

Increased emphasis in our schools on regular, sensible exercise that can be continued indefinitely in leisure time into adult life is essential if we are to remain healthy into the computer terminal age. Physicians ought to inquire into the patient's exercise habits with the same enthusiasm they bring to interrogation about current medications and bowel habits. They also should be able to refer patients with confidence to reliable information on beginning exercise and gaining access to proper facilities. Most importantly, physicians should set a good personal example, as most now do by not smoking. In the words of Cicero, "By temperance and exercise, we can preserve something of our youthful vigor, even into old age."

REFERENCES

1. Morris JN, Everitt MG, Pollard R, Chave SPW. Vigorous exercise in leisure time: protection against coronary heart disease. *Lancet* 1980;2:1207–1210.
2. Paffenbarger RS Jr, Hyde RT, Wing AL, Hsieh CC. Physical activity, all-cause mortality, and longevity of college alumni. *N Engl J Med* 1986;314:605–613.
3. Ekelund LG, Haskell WL, Johnson JL, Whaley FS, Criqui MH, Sheps DS. Physical fitness as a predictor of cardiovascular mortality in asymptomatic North American men: the Lipid Research Clinics Mortality Follow-up Study. *N Engl J Med* 1988;319:1379–1384.
4. Blair SN, Kohl HW, Paffenbarger RS, Clark DG, Cooper KH, Gibbons LW. Physical fitness and all-cause mortality. A prospective study of healthy men and women. *J Am Med Assoc* 1989;262:2395–2401.
5. Wood PD, Haskell WL, Blair SN, et al. Increased exercise level and plasma lipoprotein concentrations. A one-year, randomized, controlled study in sedentary, middle-aged men. *Metabolism* 1983;32:31–39.
6. Consensus Development Panel. *Treatment of hypertriglyceridemia.* National Institutes of Health Consensus Development Conference Summary; vol 4, no. 8, 1984.
7. Wood PD, Haskell WL, Stern MP, Lewis S, Perry C. Plasma lipoprotein distributions in male and female runners. Presented at a Conference on the Marathon, New York City, October 1976. *Ann NY Acad Sci* 1977;301:748–763.
8. Wood PDS, Stern MP, Silvers A, Reaven RM, von der Groeben J. The prevalence of plasma lipoprotein abnormalities in a free living population of the Central Valley, California. *Circulation* 1972;45:114–124.
9. Wood PD, Williams PT, Haskell WL. Physical activity and high-density lipoproteins. In: Miller NE, Miller GJ, eds. *Clinical and metabolic aspects of high-density lipoproteins.* Amsterdam: Elsevier, 1984;131–165.
10. Wood PD, Stefanick ML, Dreon DM, et al. Changes in plasma lipids and lipoproteins in overweight men during weight loss through dieting as compared with exercise. *N Engl J Med* 1988;319:1173–1179.

11. Wood PD, Stefanick ML, Haskell WL. Exercise offsets adverse lipoprotein effects of a "heart healthy" diet for weight loss [Abstract]. *Arteriosclerosis* 1989;9:773a.
12. Terry RB, Wood PD, Haskell WL, Stefanick ML, Krauss RM. Regional adiposity patterns in relation to lipids, lipoprotein cholesterol, and lipoprotein subfraction mass in men. *J Clin Endocrinol Metab* 1989;68:191–199.
13. Williams PT, Krauss RM, Wood PD, Lindgren FT, Giotas C, Vranigan KM. Lipoprotein subfractions of runners and sedentary men. *Metabolism* 1986;35:47.

Atherosclerosis Reviews, Volume 22,
edited by A. M. Gotto, Jr. and R. Paoletti.
Raven Press, Ltd., New York © 1991.

Controlling Hypertriglyceridemia in Diabetes

Antonio M. Gotto

*Department of Medicine, Baylor College of Medicine, and Internal Medicine
Service, The Methodist Hospital, Houston, Texas 77030*

There is a strong link between insulin resistance in non–insulin-dependent diabetes mellitus (NIDDM) and the development of hyperlipidemias. Hypertriglyceridemia in particular is an important risk factor for the development of coronary artery disease (CAD) and a number of other complications, foremost of which is pancreatitis (1–3). Increasing efforts have therefore been devoted to the development of appropriate antihyperlipidemic drug therapies. Because modification of lipid levels additionally reduces the hyperglycemia observed in NIDDM patients, antihyperlipidemic drugs promise to become a valuable treatment option in this condition.

Before reviewing the characteristics and uses of the principal agents in current use, the problem of diabetic hyperlipidemia and, in particular, hypertriglyceridemia will be examined.

The major indication for treating hypertriglyceridemia is to prevent the development of pancreatitis. The National Institutes of Health (NIH) Consensus Conference on Hypertriglyceridemia, held almost 10 years ago, concluded that triglyceride (TG) levels > 1,000 mg/dl require treatment owing to risk of pancreatitis, that levels > 500 mg/dl should be considered elevated, and that concentrations between 250 and 500 mg/dl are borderline. The recommendations of the National Cholesterol Education Program for evaluation and treatment of hypercholesterolemia (published in 1988), did not consider TG levels as part of the basic algorithm for treatment. Instead, their indications for treatment were based on levels of cholesterol, low-density lipoprotein (LDL) cholesterol, and a number of other risk factors. Conversely, the European guidelines for evaluating and treating hypercholesterolemia use a TG level of 200 mg/dl for separating five categories of hyperlipidemias.

There has been some debate as to whether elevation of plasma TG levels represents an independent risk for CAD, or whether it is instead a marker of some other metabolic abnormality associated with CHD. Unlike cholesterol, LDL cholesterol, and high-density lipoprotein (HDL) cholesterol, TG values do not appear to have a continuous or stepwise relationship to risk of CHD. In a number of large epidemiologic studies, TG values were associated with increased risk of CHD in univariate but not multivariate analyses (for review, see ref. 4). A difficulty with these analyses is that TG levels can be so variable. Also, TG levels tend to vary inversely with HDL levels, and the metabolism of TG-rich lipoproteins (TGRLP) is intimately tied to HDL concentrations. Analyses of data from the Framingham Study indicate that TG values are an independent risk factor for women but not for men (5). In population studies in Sweden, plasma TG concentrations were an independent risk factor for CHD (for review, see ref. 4).

Furthermore, in the recently reported Stockholm Ischemic Heart Disease Study, reduction of CHD (and of all-cause mortality) occurred only in individuals who had hypertriglyceridemia (defined as TG levels > 180 mg/dl) and who exhibited a beneficial response to treatment with nicotinic acid and clofibrate (6). In a primary intervention study, the individuals who benefited most from treatment with gemfibrozil were those who had elevations of both cholesterol and TG levels.

Hypertriglyceridemia may predispose patients to CHD owing to the atherogenicity of remnant lipoproteins, both of dietary (chylomicron remnants) and endogenous origin [LDL or very-low-density lipoprotein (VLDL) remnants]. Type III hyperlipoproteinemia is essentially a remnant disease that is associated with accelerated atherosclerosis and CHD. Most atherosclerotic plaques do not accumulate TG, whereas their cholesterol content correlates with the degree of arterial blockage.

Hypertriglyceridemia may also increase the risk for CHD by generating small, dense, apoB-enriched LDL particles. A similar process is thought to occur in the formation of these LDL particles as in the formation of small HDL particles. Thus, an LDL fraction is generated from TGRLP, which is then converted by hepatic TG lipase to small apoB-enriched LDL particles. Increased atherogenicity of these latter particles is assumed, but it has not been conclusively demonstrated.

There should be less question about treating hypertriglyceridemia in the diabetic patient than in the nondiabetic. The same risk factors operate for CHD and pancreatitis in the diabetic as in the nondiabetic. Also, the diabetic patient has a further increase in risk owing to the presence of diabetes.

The first step in the treatment of hypertriglyceridemia in the diabetic is to make sure that the diabetes is under adequate control, because this condition may be secondary to poorly controlled diabetes. Hyperinsulinemia, resulting from insulin resistance in NIDDM, may cause excessive synthesis of VLDL by the liver, with hyperlipidemia as a consequence. The physician should use the usual parameters, such as fasting and postprandial glucose levels and concentrations of glycosylated hemoglobin, to determine the adequacy of diabetic control. If the diabetes is not adequately controlled, the choice of therapy must be reconsidered.

In the NIDDM patient, control of obesity is of utmost importance. In general, control of obesity and decrease of alcohol consumption are the two cornerstones for controlling hypertriglyceridemia. In addition, exercise decreases plasma TG concentrations both in itself and by serving as an adjunct to weight control. If the patient is receiving oral hypoglycemic therapy, the dose may need to be adjusted.

Having established the best possible control of the patient's diabetes, it is then appropriate to reevaluate the plasma TG levels. If improved diabetic control has corrected hypertriglyceridemia, it is reasonable to assume that it was secondary to the diabetes. In some cases, inherited forms of hypertriglyceridemia are associated with diabetes. This is particularly true in mixed hypertriglyceridemia, or type V hyperlipidemia, which is associated with fasting chylomicronemia, glucose intolerance, hyperuricemia and episodes of abdominal pain, and pancreatitis.

If meticulous control of diabetes and nonpharmacologic measures are insufficient, and the TG level remains > 250 mg/dl, then drug therapy should be considered. The drug used should depend on the primary pattern of hyperlipidemia. Diabetics may have the same pattern of signs and symptoms seen in nondiabetics, but hypertriglyceridemia with increased VLDL levels is particularly common, and chylomicronemia may also accompany the increase in VLDL levels in patients with type V hyperlipidemia.

Currently, the most commonly used drugs for the treatment of hyperlipidemias are the fibric acid derivative gemfibrozil and nicotinic acid (7,8). The principal action of nicotinic acid is to inhibit the release of free fatty acids from adipocytes. In addition, it blocks the lipolytic actions of a number of endogenous mediators such as glucagon, catecholamines, corticotropin, growth hormone, and glucocorticoids, by inhibiting activation of the lipase enzyme. Nicotinic acid is metabolized in the liver by conjugation with glycine—a reaction that utilizes acetyl CoA. The diversion of acetyl CoA from cholesterol synthesis may explain the reported inhibition of cholesterol synthesis at the pre–mevalonic acid stage by this agent.

Use of nicotinic acid, however, is associated with a number of adverse side effects. One problem is that in some diabetics, this drug worsens glucose intolerance. Furthermore, it is necessary to use relatively high doses of the drug—3 to 4.5 g/day. Virtually all patients experience flushing with this agent. Other side effects including dizziness, palpitations, and pruritis. Nicotinic acid therapy must be started at low doses—for example, 100 mg with a meal—and gradually increased over a period of weeks until a maintenance dose is reached.

Newer analogues of nicotinic acid, with fewer side effects, have been developed. These agents, such as acipimox (5-methylpyrazine carboxylic acid-4-oxide), are more suitable for long-term use in NIDDM patients. The principal action of acipimox is to inhibit the hormone-sensitive lipase of lipoid tissues and the hepatic lipase enzyme. This action decreases lipolysis; as a result, plasma TG and VLDL levels are reduced. Acipimox also decreases hepatic HDL catabolism, thereby raising plasma HDL levels. A further beneficial effect of lowering plasma TG levels in NIDDM patients is an increase in glucose uptake and utilization by the tissues, hence reducing hyperglycemia.

Gemfibrozil, an isobutyric acid derivative, has been shown to reduce plasma levels of TG, cholesterol, LDL, and VLDL, while raising HDL concentrations (9). Its effects on TG levels may be mediated through inhibition of hepatic VLDL synthesis and an increase in plasma VLDL clearance.

In some patients with hypertriglyceridemia, fibric acid derivatives may cause a small increase in LDL cholesterol levels. If a patient has mild hypertriglyceridemia but substantially increased LDL levels, the use of an HMG-CoA reductase inhibitor such as lovastatin may be considered. Lovastatin is a competitive inhibitor of 3-hydroxy-3-methylglutaryl coenzyme A reductase (HMG-CoA reductase), which is the rate-determining enzyme in cholesterol synthesis. Thus, plasma cholesterol and LDL levels are reduced, with either a slight increase or no effect upon plasma HDL levels. Recently, excellent responses to lovastatin in terms of LDL reduction have been described in NIDDM patients.

In summary, it is very important to manage elevated TG levels in the diabetic. The first step is to determine if the elevation is due to poor control of diabetes. If diabetic control is adequate and hypertriglyceridemia persists, diet and exercise are the first line of therapy, followed by use of a lipid-lowering agent.

REFERENCES

1. American Diabetes Association. Role of cardiovascular risk factors in prevention and treatment of macrovascular disease in diabetes. *Diabetes Care* 1989;12:573–579.
2. Barrett-Connor E, Orchard T. Diabetes and heart disease. In: National Diabetes Data Group. *Diabetes in America: diabetes data compiled 1984*. Washington, D.C.: U.S. Dept. of Health and Human Services; 1985:Chap. 16. (National Institutes of Health publication 85-1468.)
3. Uusitupa M, Niskanen LK, Siitonen O, et al. Five-Year Incidence of atherosclerotic vascular disease in relation to general risk factors, insulin level, and abnormalities in lipoprotein composition in non–insulin-dependent diabetic and nondiabetic subjects. *Circulation* 1990;82:27–36.
4. Austin MA. Plasma triglyceride and coronary heart disease. *Arterioscleros Thromb* 1991;11:2–14.
5. Kannel WB. Metabolic risk factors for coronary heart disease in women: perspective from the Framingham Study. *Am Heart J* 1987;114:413–419.
6. Clarson LA, Rosenhamer G. Reduction of mortality in the Stockholm Ischaemic Heart Disease Secondary Prevention Study by combined treatment with clofibrate and nicotinic acid. *Acta Med Scand* 1988;223:405–418.
7. Garg A, Grundy SM. Gemfibrozil alone and in combination with lovastatin for treatment of hypertriglyceridemia in NIDDM. *Diabetes* 1989;38:364–372.
8. Garg A, Grundy SM. Nicotinic acid as therapy for dyslipidemia in non-insulin-dependent diabetes mellitus. *JAMA* 1990;264:723–726.
9. Manninen V, Elo MO, Frick MH, et al. Lipid alterations and decline in the incidence of coronary heart disease in the Helsinki Heart Study. *JAMA* 1988;260:641–651.

Atherosclerosis Reviews, Volume 22,
edited by A. M. Gotto, Jr. and R. Paoletti.
Raven Press, Ltd., New York © 1991.

The Glucose–Fatty Acid Cycle

Biochemical Aspects

Philip J. Randle

*Nuffield Department of Clinical Biochemistry, University of Oxford, John
Radcliffe Hospital, Oxford OX3 9DU, England*

The departure in thought that formed the basis of the concept of a glucose–
fatty acid cycle in 1963 was the idea that the relationship between the utilization of glucose and lipid fuels in energy metabolism is reciprocal and not
dependent. In 1956, when the work began, the prevailing concept was that
the oxidation of lipid fuels [free fatty acids (FFA) and ketone bodies (KB)]
is a passive consequence of diminished glucose utilization in, for example,
starvation or uncontrolled diabetes. The new concept was prompted by the
discovery of lipolysis as a glucose-independent process, directly modulated
by hormones such as epinephrine and insulin, and by the discovery that FFA
and KB inhibit glucose uptake, glycolysis, and oxidation of glucose (pyruvate) in rat heart and diaphragm muscles. In the late 1960s, doubts as to its
general applicability were raised when a number of investigations failed to
show inhibitory effects of lipid fuels on glucose utilization in skeletal muscle
preparations. However, these doubts were largely dispelled by a series of
papers from 1975 onward which confirmed that FFA and/or KB inhibit glucose utilization in a variety of *in vitro* preparations of red skeletal muscle.
These aspects are reviewed in (1,2). From the point of view of the role of
triglycerides in disease processes, the major interest is in the effects that
FFA may have on carbohydrate metabolism in humans in relation to hypertriglyceridemia and non–insulin-dependent diabetes mellitus (NIDDM).

EFFECTS OF FFA AND NIDDM ON CARBOHYRDATE METABOLISM IN HUMANS

The major disturbances of carbohydrate metabolism in NIDDM are enhanced glucose production in the postabsorptive state and impaired glucose
utilization (storage and oxidation) following intake of glucose (3–5). Storage
(mainly glycogen synthesis) is quantitatively greater than oxidation except
at low intakes. There is insulin resistance in regard to these parameters (3–

5) as well as modest hypoinsulinemia (6). The major site of insulin resistance is extrahepatic, predominantly in skeletal muscles. There is also insulin resistance with regard to release and oxidation of FFA (4).

In normal people, acute elevation of plasma FFA by administration of triglyceride (TG) plus heparin decreases total glucose uptake, glucose oxidation, and nonoxidative glucose disposal (glucose storage) by 20% to 55%. It also increases FFA oxidation 1.5- to 6-fold and induces insulin resistance with regard to these parameters (7,8).

SHORTER-TERM REGULATORY MECHANISMS IN THE GLUCOSE–FATTY ACID CYCLE

The phrase "shorter-term regulatory mechanisms" is used to describe changes readily demonstrable within a matter of minutes with *in vitro* rat or mouse tissue preparations or within seconds with isolated enzymes. They are based mainly on allosteric transition or reversible phosphorylation. Longer-term regulatory mechanisms require hours and are based mainly on altered rates of gene expression.

Fatty Acid Oxidation

The major determinant of fatty acid oxidation is the rate of lipolysis of adipocyte triglyceride (TG). This is determined by the activity of hormone-sensitive lipase, which is switched on through phosphorylation by cyclic AMP (cAMP) kinase (and hence by hormones that increase cAMP concentration) and switched off by insulin through two mechanisms—activation of a protein phosphatase and activation of cAMP phosphodiesterase (Fig. 1). In rat models of diabetes or starvation and in NIDDM in humans, TG is deposited in muscle and lipolyzed by hormone-sensitive lipase. Deposition of TG is associated with insulin resistance in rat muscle (9). Lipolysis of circulating TG by lipoprotein lipase may be important in NIDDM and is used experimentally as a means of acutely raising plasma FFA in normal people.

Glucose Oxidation and Glycolysis

Glucose oxidation rate is determined by the activity of the mitochondrial pyruvate dehydrogenase (PDH) complex, which is regulated mainly by reversible phosphorylation (phosphorylation being inactivating) (Fig. 2). Activity of PDH complex is determined by the proportion in the active form—i.e., by the relative activities of PDH kinase and PDH phosphatase. Shorter-term regulation of PDH kinase is mainly effected by end products common to PDH complex and FFA oxidation (acetyl CoA and NADH) through the

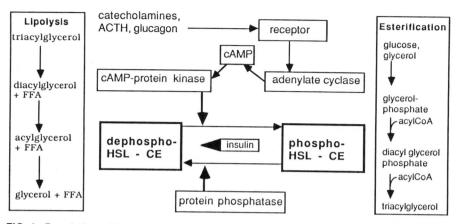

FIG. 1. Regulation of lipolysis by hormone sensitive lipase/cholesterol esterase (HSL-CE).

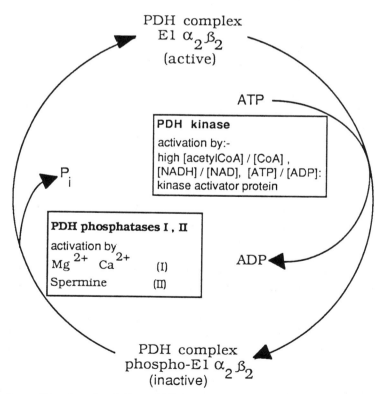

FIG. 2. Reversible phosphorylation of PDH complex and regulation of PDH kinase and phosphatase.

concentration ratios (acetyl CoA)/(CoA) and (NADH)/(NAD). Increases in these ratios accompany the oxidation of lipid fuels and mediate their effects to decrease the percentage of PDH$_a$. PDH phosphatase is regulated by Ca^{2+} ions (which mediate effects of exercise and of Ca^{2+} signaling of hormone action) to increase the percentage of PDH$_a$. Insulin activates PDH phosphatase and increases the percent of PDH$_a$ in adipocytes and possibly liver by an unknown mechanism; it has no such effect in muscles. These mechanisms of regulation apply to human PDH complex.

When PDH complex is inactivated in the course of the oxidation of lipid fuels, glycolysis is inhibited in parallel through inhibition of PFK1 by citrate (and in liver by lowering of fructose 2.6 bisphosphate through inhibition of PFK2 by citrate). This coupled regulation of pyruvate oxidation (PDH complex) and pyruvate formation (glycolysis) serves to prevent the excessive lactate accumulation that would otherwise occur. It also leads (through inhibition of glucose phosphorylation) to inhibition of glucose uptake.

Other Aspects of Glucose Metabolism

In heart muscle, the effect of low (physiological) concentrations of insulin to stimulate glucose transport is inhibited by lipid fuels—i.e., they induce insulin resistance. There is published evidence for a comparable effect in rat diaphragm muscle but not in rat soleus muscle. The effect of elevation of plasma FFA to inhibit glucose storage (presumably glycogen synthesis) in humans has not been studied in skeletal muscle *in vitro*. This is of some importance because *in vivo* effects of TG plus heparin are only reliably ascribed to effects of FFA when mechanisms are clear.

LONGER-TERM REGULATORY MECHANISMS

Studies in rat models have shown that the effects of starvation or alloxan diabetes to decrease the percent of PDH$_a$ in muscles and liver cannot be explained wholly by shorter-term effects of FFA oxidation to activate PDH kinase. It was shown in these models that starvation and diabetes produce a stable increase in the activity of PDH kinase by a longer-term mechanism requiring 24 hr to 48 hr. In studies in tissue culture with hepatocytes or cardiac myocytes from normal rats, it has been shown that this effect of starvation or diabetes can be reproduced by 24 hr of exposure to FFA or analogues of cAMP [see (1,2)]. The mechanism is not yet fully defined; it may involve an increase in PDH kinase or increased activity of a protein activator of PDH kinase (see Fig. 3). The observation is extremely important because it shows longer-term effects of FFA and cAMP; on glucose oxidation; it shows parallelism between the effects of FFA and cAMP; it emphasizes the need for studies of longer-term effects of FFA in humans *in*

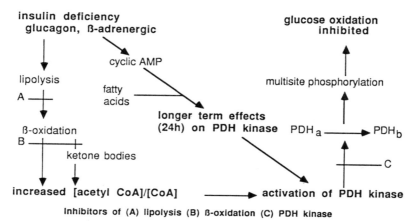

FIG. 3. Mechanisms mediating effects of starvation and diabetes to enhance phosphorylation and inactivation of PDH complex in rat tissues.

vivo; and it suggests the need to search for other parallel and longer-term effects of cAMP and FFA—e.g., on the insulin receptor and its tyrosine kinase.

THE GLUCOSE FATTY ACID CYCLE: LIPOLYSIS AND HUMAN DIABETES

The parallelism between effects of NIDDM and of acute elevation of plasma FFA in normal people on the rate and pattern of glucose disposal and on insulin sensitivity does no more than suggest that FFA may have a role in the disturbed glucose metabolism and insulin sensitivity of diabetics. However, drugs that act as inhibitors of lipolysis (e.g., acipimox) or of FFA oxidation (e.g., methyl palmoxirate) or of PDH kinase (e.g., dichloroacetate) promote glucose utilization and oxidation in NIDDM (and IDDM) patients and are hypoglycemic. The evidence overall suffices to show that fatty acid oxidation inhibits glucose oxidation in humans and that fatty acid oxidation contributes to inhibition of glucose oxidation in NIDDM and IDDM. The results with dichloroacetate indicate that the mechanism involves PDH kinase and reversible phosphorylation in the PDH complex, but it has yet to be confirmed by direct measurements of percent of PDH$_a$. The value of published negative findings in biopsy samples of human muscle is uncertain because of known technical problems with such measurements in skeletal muscle. The contribution of FFA oxidation to impaired glucose storage and insulin resistance in NIDDM is less certain. Acipimox improves oxidative and nonoxidative disposal of glucose and insulin sensitivity in NIDDM, but there is no clear evidence that this is secondary to inhibition of lipolysis and of FFA oxidation. If acipimox is antilipolytic through an effect on adipocyte cAMP (or cAMP kinase), then it may well activate glycogen synthesis in muscle by direct effects on cAMP (or cAMP kinase) in muscle. Phosphorylation by cAMP kinase inhibits muscle glycogen synthase.

Note added in proof: Since this review was written, it has been shown that the longer term increase in the activity of PDH kinase induced in rats by diabetes or starvation is due to an increase of the activity of PDH kinase *per se* and not to a protein activator. [Mistry SC, Priestman DA, Kerbey AL, Randle PJ. *Biochem J* 1991;275 (in press).]

REFERENCES

1. Randle PJ. *Biochem Soc Trans* 1986;14:799–806.
2. Randle PJ, Kerbey AL, Espinal J. *Diabetes/Metab Rev* 1988;4:623–638.
3. Meyer HV, Curchod B, Maeder E, Pahud P, Jequier E, Felber P. *Diabetes* 1986;31:957–963.
4. Groop RC, Bonadonna RC, Delprato S, et al. *J Clin Invest* 1989;84:205–213.
5. Shulman GI, Rothman DL, Jue T, Stein P, DeFronzo RA, Shulman RG. *N Engl J Med* 1990;322:223–228.
6. Temple RC, Carrington CA, Lazio SD, et al. *Lancet* 1989;1:293–295.
7. Schalch DS, Kipnis DM. *J Clin Invest* 1965;44:2010–2020.
8. Thiebaud D, DeFronzo RA, Jacot E, et al. *Metabolism* 1982;31:1128–1136.
9. Denton RM, Randle PJ. Biochem J 1967;104:416–422.
10. Jenkins AB, Storlein LH, Pascoe WS, Chisholm DJ, Kraegen EW. Presented at Internation Symposium "Triglyceride—the Role in Diabetes and Atherosclerosis," Vienna, May 1990.
11. Fulcher GR, Walker M, Sum CF, et al. Presented at International Symposium "Triglyceride—the Role in Diabetes and Atherosclerosis," Vienna, May 1990.

Atherosclerosis Reviews, Volume 22,
edited by A. M. Gotto, Jr. and R. Paoletti.
Raven Press, Ltd., New York © 1991.

Molecular Basis for the Randle Hypothesis in Patients with Non–Insulin-Dependent Diabetes Mellitus

Allan Vaag and Henning Beck-Nielsen

Department of Internal Medicine M, Odense University Hospital,
5000 Odense C, Denmark

Patients with non–insulin-dependent diabetes mellitus (NIDDM) are characterized by resistance to insulin-stimulated glucose uptake in skeletal muscles; and it is generally believed that this defect plays an important role in the pathogenesis of the syndrome. Patients with NIDDM often have elevated concentrations of nonesterified fatty acids (NEFA) in plasma. Furthermore, elevations in plasma NEFA concentration have been shown to lower insulin-stimulated glucose uptake in normal individuals. Thus, it has been hypothesized that insulin resistance in patients with NIDDM may be caused by—or at least be due in part to—elevated NEFA concentrations in plasma.

We do not fully understand the mechanisms that control the relationship between fatty acid and glucose utilization in human skeletal muscle. The classical glucose–fatty acid cycle, demonstrated by Randle et al. (1) in isolated rat hearts and hemidiaphragms, involves an inhibitory effect of NEFA on glycolysis and pyruvate oxidation. In this model, no effect of NEFA on glycogen synthesis was demonstrated. The same group showed that the inhibitory effect of NEFA on glycolysis and glucose oxidation was caused by a build-up of mitochondrial citrate and acetyl coenzyme A (CoA), and a rise in the cytoplasmic NADH/NAD ratio. Citrate inhibits the activity of phosphofructokinase (PFK), which may be the main rate regulating enzymatic step in the glycolysis; and acetyl CoA inhibits the activity of pyruvate dehydrogenase (PDH), which is thought to represent the rate-determining enzymatic step in the oxidation of glucose.

Acipimox is a long-acting antilipolytic nicotinic acid analogue that greatly lowers plasma concentrations of NEFA. The aim of this study was to evaluate the effect of inhibition of lipolysis with acipimox on glucose metabolism in patients with NIDDM. By taking biopsy samples from skeletal muscles, we hoped to elucidate whether changes in key enzyme activities in this tissue could be responsible for any of the *in vivo* effects of acipimox.

The acute effect of acipimox (2×250 mg) on basal and insulin-stimulated (40 mU/m^2/min) glucose metabolism was therefore studied in 12 patients with NIDDM in a double-blind cross-over study. Basal hyperglycemia was maintained during insulin stimulation (isoglycemic clamp procedure) and whole-body glucose metabolism was assessed using 3-[^{3}H]glucose and indirect calorimetry. Biopsy samples were taken from the vastus lateralis muscle during basal and insulin-stimulated steady-state periods. Acipimox reduced NEFA in the basal state (0.12 ± 0.02 versus 0.70 ± 0.05 mM; $p < 0.01$) and during insulin stimulation (0.05 ± 0.01 versus 0.09 ± 0.01 mM; $p < 0.05$). Lipid oxidation was inhibited by acipimox in all patients in the basal state (20 ± 2 versus 33 ± 3 mg/m^2/min; $p < 0.01$) and during insulin infusion (8 ± 2 versus 17 ± 2 mg/m^2/min; $p < 0.01$). Total glucose turnover (Rd) was unaffected by acipimox in the basal state (97 ± 3 versus 94 ± 4 mg/m^2/min); whereas during insulin infusion, acipimox increased Rd (372 ± 49 versus 262 ± 31 mg/m^2/min; $p < 0.01$). Acipimox increased glucose oxidation in the basal state (76 ± 4 versus 50 ± 4 mg/m^2/min; $p < 0.01$). During insulin stimulation, acipimox increased both glucose oxidation (121 ± 7 versus 95 ± 4 mg/m^2/min; $p < 0.01$) and nonoxidative glucose disposal (251 ± 47 versus 167 ± 29 mg/m^2/min; $p < 0.01$). Acipimox enhanced the basal and insulin-stimulated activity of glycogen synthase (GS) in muscle biopsy specimens [fractional velocity (0.1 and 10 mM G-6-P) = 31 ± 2 versus $25 \pm 3\%$; $p < 0.05$, and 50 ± 5 versus $41 \pm 4\%$; $p < 0.05$]. Activities of PDH and PFK in muscle biopsy specimens were unaffected by acipimox.

In conclusion, acipimox acutely improves insulin action in patients with NIDDM by increasing both glucose oxidation and nonoxidative glucose disposal. This finding supports the hypothesis that elevated NEFA is important for insulin resistance in NIDDM. Furthermore, these results demonstrate that the glucose–fatty acid cycle (Randle cycle) operates in patients with NIDDM on a whole-body basis. The mechanism responsible for the increased insulin-stimulated nonoxidative glucose disposal may be a stimulatory effect of acipimox on glycogen synthase activity in skeletal muscles. Increased activities of PDH and PFK in skeletal muscles may not be responsible for the effect of acipimox on whole-body glucose oxidation. This fact would suggest that skeletal muscles are not responsible for the effect of acipimox on whole-body glucose oxidation or, alternatively, that the biochemical mechanisms that control the interaction between fatty acid and glucose metabolism in human skeletal muscles may be different from the mechanisms pointed out by Randle et al. (1) in perfused rat hearts and hemidiaphragms.

A long-term study with acipimox is needed to demonstrate whether the acute beneficial effect on glucose metabolism can also lead to long-term improvement of metabolic control in NIDDM patients.

REFERENCES

1. Randle PJ, Garland PB, Hales CN, Newsholme EA. The glucose fatty-acid cycle: its role in insulin sensitivity and the metabolic disturbances of diabetes mellitus. *Lancet* 1963;1:785–787.

Atherosclerosis Reviews, Volume 22,
edited by A. M. Gotto, Jr. and R. Paoletti.
Raven Press, Ltd., New York © 1991.

Metabolic Effects of Acipimox in Non–Insulin-Dependent Diabetes Mellitus

K. G. M. M. Alberti, G. Fulcher, and M. Walker

*Department of Medicine, The Medical School,
Newcastle upon Tyne NE2 4HH, England*

Non–insulin-dependent diabetes mellitus (NIDMM) is a common disorder found in every country in the world. Prevalence varies from < 1% to > 20% in certain special groups. It is characterized by defects in both insulin secretion and insulin action. Among the major defects that result in the pathognomonic hyperglycemia of the syndrome are: (a) increased hepatic glucose output, causing fasting hyperglycemia; (b) decreased insulin-mediated glucose uptake in peripheral tissues, primarily muscle, which causes postprandial hyperglycemia; and (c) inappropriately elevated plasma nonesterified fatty acid (NEFA) levels. The NEFA levels are of particular interest, because it is conceivable that they play a role in the first two defects.

Many years ago, Randle et al. (1) postulated that fatty acids could inhibit glucose oxidation in rat muscle secondary to the inhibition of glucose phosphorylation and the phosphofructokinase (PFK) and pyruvate dehydogenase (PDH) reactions. They suggested that there was a glucose–fatty acid cycle that caused decreased glucose utilization when fatty acid levels were high and increased glucose utilization when levels were low. Subsequently, others have shown *in vivo* in humans that even modest elevations of fatty acid levels decrease insulin-stimulated glucose clearance by muscle (2,3). Fatty acid oxidation also drives gluconeogenesis in the liver (4). It is thus attractive to speculate that lowering fatty acid levels might improve glucose utilization, decrease hepatic glucose output, and hence lower blood glucose levels in diabetic humans. One obvious approach to investigating this issue is to inhibit lipolysis, thus cutting off NEFA supplies to both liver and muscle.

An inhibitor of lipolysis, nicotinic acid, has been available for use in humans for many years; indeed it has been freely used as a hypolipidemic agent. It has, however, been contraindicated in NIDDM, because it has been shown to worsen glucose tolerance (5). Close examination of the data shows that it has a short duration of action with considerable rebound in NEFA, which matches glucose levels closely. More recently, a nicotinic acid derivative, acipimox, has become available. Acipimox has many fewer side effects and a longer duration of action (6); therefore, we conducted a series of studies using acipimox to inhibit lipolysis in order to establish the metabolic effects on glucose metabolism of lowering NEFA in NIDDM. These studies have been acute, subacute, and chronic; they are described briefly below.

ACUTE STUDIES WITH ACIPIMOX

The first studies were performed to examine the effect of a small dose of acipimox (250 mg) on glucose tolerance and insulin sensitivity. Acipimox or placebo was given to NIDDM subjects after an overnight fast. Two hours later, either a 75-g oral glucose load or a 150-min glucose–insulin infusion (0.05 U/kg/hr insulin plus 6 mg/kg/min glucose) were given. In both cases, by the start of the test plasma NEFA levels were suppressed to almost zero at the beginning of the appropriate test. Oral glucose tolerance was significantly improved by acipimox.

In the glucose-insulin infusion test, blood glucose is measured from 120 min to 150 min after the start of the infusion, and the mean blood glucose gives a measure of insulin sensitivity (7). The lower the glucose, the greater the insulin sensitivity. In the placebo study, the mean final blood glucose was 9.0 ± 1.0 mmol/L; whereas after acipimox, the value was 7.1 ± 0.8 mmol/L. Thus, acutely at least, acipimox appeared to improve both glucose tolerance and insulin sensitivity.

OVERNIGHT STUDIES WITH ACIPIMOX

A major problem in NIDDM is fasting hyperglycemia, which represents increased hepatic glucose production in the overnight period. We therefore conducted a series of overnight studies with acipimox in NIDDM subjects. In the first study, 250 mg was given immediately preceding the evening meal. Plasma NEFA were immediately suppressed, reaching a nadir of 0.06 mmol/L after 3 hr. By 8 hr, however, values had returned to baseline and were indistinguishable from those found after placebo. Blood glucose levels were lower with the drug than with the placebo both during the evening meal and throughout the night. Overall, the mean overnight glucose was 12% lower with acipimox, although values were not significantly different by next morning. In addition, glucose turnover was not different next morning. Thus, the effect of acipimox was too short to last overnight.

In a second overnight study, obese NIDDM subjects were given 250 mg acipimox (or placebo) at 1900 hr before dinner, at 0100, and at 0600 hr. This resulted in NEFA suppression throughout the night, with levels of 0.11 ± 0.02 mmol/L versus 0.65 mmol/L on placebo at 0800 hr. Ketone body (KB) levels were similarly depressed. Fasting blood glucose levels were decreased in the acipimox group (8.3 versus 9.8 mmol/L) as was hepatic glucose production (2.04 ± 0.18 mg/kg/min versus 2.58 mg/kg/min). A euglycemic hyperinsulinemic clamp was performed. During this time, glucose clearance was enhanced by 33% in the low NEFA patients, and hepatic glucose output was more fully inhibited. Patients also underwent indirect calorimetry both before and at the end of the clamp. This procedure led to a doubling of glucose oxidation and a halving of lipid oxidation in the basal state and similar changes at the end of the clamp.

A further acute experiment was undertaken to examine whether acipimox was exerting any effects independently of the decrease in circulating NEFA levels. Normal subjects were studied. They were given acipimox or placebo at 0 and 90 min and a euglycemic clamp was performed from 120 min to 240 min, together with infusion of 10% Intralipid (25 ml/hr) and heparin (0.4 U/kg/hr) for 4 hr from time zero. Plasma NEFA levels were similar on placebo and acipimox at the beginning and end of the clamp (0.48 ± 0.05 mmol/L, acipimox; 0.51 ± 0.10 mmol/L, placebo, at end of clamp). 3-Hydroxybutyrate and triglyceride (TG) levels were also similar on control and drug days. Nevertheless, there was significantly greater glucose infusion to maintain euglycemia during the clamp when acipimox was given, implying greater insulin sensitivity. Carbohydrate oxidation was, however, unaffected; therefore, the increase must all be accounted for by a 20% increase in glucose storage as glycogen.

We concluded from these various studies that lowering NEFA levels did indeed increase glucose disposal, mainly through oxidation, and decrease hepatic glucose output. This process resulted in a significant, although modest, fall in blood glucose levels. In addition, acipimox itself appears to have a fatty acid independent effect, increasing glycogen storage. This action could be a direct effect on glycogen synthase; an effect on glucose transport; or, alternatively, an effect mediated through changes in intramuscular TG.

CHRONIC ADMINISTRATION OF ACIPIMOX

Although acute studies are of value in investigating mechanisms, longer-term studies are essential to establish whether a drug is of therapeutic use. We therefore performed a double-blind cross-over study of acipimox (250 mg t.i.d.) versus placebo in patients with NIDDM, using 3-month treatment periods with a washout period in between arms of the study. Patients on acipimox showed the expected improvement in serum cholesterol and TG levels. There was also a small decrease in plasma NEFA levels. Although acutely there was an improvement in insulin sensitivity, there were no changes in parameters reflecting overall glycemic control.

These results could perhaps be predicted from the known pharmacodynamics of acipimox. Thus the studies described earlier clearly show that when given on a three-times-daily basis, the drug cannot give 24-hr suppression of lipolysis. In addition, other investigators have suggested that clinically, administration of the drug results in periods of suppression interspersed with rebounds in NEFA levels. This rebound effect is particularly relevant in the overnight period. It should be emphasized, however, that by contrast with nicotinic acid, control of the condition did not worsen.

The obvious solution is to find a longer-acting formulation of the drug. We have already begun preliminary studies with such a preparation, and the results are encouraging. There is clear evidence that the drug remains effective for 10 hr, although not for 12 hr. It will, however, allow for overnight suppression of lipolysis.

CONCLUSIONS

NIDDM is characterized by insulin resistance and increased hepatic glucose production. These conditions can be modified, at least acutely, by decreasing circulatory fatty acid levels with agents such as acipimox. Acipimox also improves lipid levels in diabetic patients, causing a fall in TG and low-density lipoprotein cholesterol and an increase in high-density lipoprotein cholesterol. The drug would obviously have therapeutic appeal if it could be shown to improve glycemic control as well. This action has not proved consistently possible so far, presumably because of the short duration of action of the drug. Preliminary studies with a longer-acting preparation are, however, encouraging. At present, acipimox can be used safely in diabetic patients as a hypolipidemic agent, and in the future, it may also be useful in improving glycemic control.

REFERENCES

1. Randle PJ, Hales CN, Garland PB, Newsholme EA. The glucose–fatty acid cycle. Its role in insulin sensitivity and the metabolic disturbances of diabetes mellitus. *Lancet* 1963;1:785–789.
2. Ferrannini E, Barrett EJ, Bevilaqua S, DeFronzo RA. Effect of fatty acid on glucose production and utilization in man. *J Clin Invest* 1983;72:1737–1747.
3. Walker M, Fulcher GR, Catalano C. Physiological levels of non-esterified fatty acids impair forearm glucose uptake in normal man [Abstract]. *Diabetologia* 1989;32:555.
4. Blumenthal SA. Stimulation of gluconeogenesis by palmitic acid in rat hepatocytes: evidence that this effect can be dissociated from provision of reducing equivalents. *Metabolism* 1983;32:971–976.
5. Carlson LA, Ostman J. Inhibition of the mobilisation of free fatty acids from adipose tissue in diabetes. II. Effect of nicotinic acid and acetylsalicylate on blood glucose in human diabetics. *Acta Med Scand* 1965;178:71–79.
6. Fucella LM, Goldaniga G, Lovislo P, et al. Inhibition of lipolysis by nicotinic acid and by acipimox. *Clin Pharmacol Ther* 1980;28:790–795.
7. Heine RJ, Home PD, Ponchner M, et al. A comparison of three methods for assessing insulin sensitivity in subjects with normal and abnormal glucose tolerance. *Diabetes Res* 1985;2:113–120.

Atherosclerosis Reviews, Volume 22,
edited by A. M. Gotto, Jr. and R. Paoletti.
Raven Press, Ltd., New York © 1991.

Nicotinic Acid and Acipimox

Similarities and Differences

Göran Walldius and Per Tornvall

*Karolinska Hospital and King Gustaf V Research Institute,
S-104 01 Stockholm, Sweden*

Nicotinic acid is an effective lipid-lowering agent. The use of nicotinic acid in the treatment of hyperlipoproteinemia is often limited by the frequent occurrence of side effects. Flushing, pruritis, diarrhea, nausea, flatulence, elevation of liver transaminases, hyperglycemia, and abnormal glucose tolerance have been reported in many nondiabetic patients taking nicotinic acid (1). Acipimox (Farmitalia Carlo Erba, Italy), a nicotinic acid analogue (5-methyl-pyrazine-carboxylic acid 4-oxide), lowers blood lipids effectively (2). Acipimox causes few side effects and does not appear to impair glucose homeostasis (3).

Therefore, we decided to compare the effects of acipimox and nicotinic acid on serum lipids and lipoproteins and on glucose metabolism. The drugs were also compared in regard to tolerability and side effects. Our subjects were nondiabetic patients with hypertriglyceridemia.

MATERIALS AND METHODS

Twenty nondiabetic, asymptomatic hyperlipidemic patients (13 type IV, 6 type IIB, and 1 type III), aged 42 to 68 years (mean age, 51 years) were treated for 6 weeks with acipimox 250 mg t.i.d. and nicotinic acid 1 gm t.i.d. according to an open, randomized cross-over design. Side effects during the treatment periods were evaluated by questionnaire. A subjective scoring system was used.

PRELIMINARY RESULTS

Serum Lipids

Average pretreatment serum triglyceride (TG) levels in the two groups were 5.6 mmol/L and 5.2 mmol/L, respectively. The corresponding cholesterol values were 9.0 mmol/L and 8.4 mmol/L. Differences in lipid values between groups were not significant. Cholesterol was decreased by 12% by both drugs (acipimox $p < 0.05$, nicotinic acid $p < 0.001$). Triglycerides were decreased by 27% with acipimox and by 36% with nicotinic acid ($p < 0.001$). Very-low-density lipoproteins (VLDL) were decreased by about 40% ($p < 0.001$). High-density lipoproteins (HDL) were increased by about 15% by both treatments (acipimox $p < 0.001$, nicotinic acid $p < 0.001$). Neither drug affected low-density lipoprotein (LDL) levels. The effects of nicotinic acid and acipimox on lipid parameters were not significantly different between the two groups.

Glucose Metabolism

Average pretreatment fasting blood glucose levels in the two groups were 5.5 mmol/L and 5.5 mmol/L, respectively. The blood glucose response to a 75-g oral glucose load was not modified by acipimox ($0'-30'-60'-90'-120'$ values were 5.5, 9.0, 10.4, 10.0, 8.4 mmol/L pretreatment and 5.4, 8.9, 10.4, 10.2, 8.6 mmol/L posttreatment). However, nicotinic acid significantly increased blood glucose after 90 min ($p < 0.005$; corresponding values were 5.6, 8.7, 10.2, 9.2, 8.2, mmol/L pretreatment and 5.8, 9.0, 10.8, 10.7, 8.7 mmol/L posttreatment).

Side Effects

According to a subjective scoring system on a questionnaire filled in by the patient, flushing and pruritis occurred for a significantly greater length of time ($p < 0.001$) and with significantly greater severity ($p < 0.001$) in the patients receiving nicotinic acid as compared to those receiving acipimox.

DISCUSSION

Acipimox and nicotinic acid appear to have about similar effects on blood lipid parameters. We could find no significant differences between the two treatment groups in efficacy of reducing serum cholesterol and TG or of increasing HDL cholesterol levels.

Nicotinic acid increased blood glucose levels significantly during the oral glucose load. Acipimox, however, had no or little effect on glucose metabolism. Acipimox appears to be a good alternative to nicotinic acid, as many patients with hypertriglyceridemia have borderline or elevated fasting glucose levels. These patients often develop type II diabetes later in life. It appears that the risk of developing adult-onset diabetes is reduced more effectively with acipimox therapy than with nicotinic acid therapy, but further research in this area is required.

Our results indicate that the side effects of acipimox therapy are less severe and of shorter duration than the side effects of nicotinic acid. Acipimox appears to be safer and less toxic than nicotinic acid while at the same time being a comparably effective lipid-lowering agent. We are now preparing a final report based on a larger population sample.

REFERENCES

1. Walldius G, Wahlberg G. Effects of nicotinic acid and its derivatives on lipid metabolism and other metabolic factors related to atherosclerosis. In: Kritchensky D, Holmes WL, Paoletti R, eds. *Drugs affecting lipid metabolism* VIII. Plenum New York: 1985;281–293.
2. Crepaldi G, Avogaro P, Deseovich GC, et al. Plasma lipid lowering activity of acipimox in patients with type II and type IV hyperlipoproteinemia. *Atherosclerosis* 1988;70:115–121.
3. Lavezzari M, Milanesi G, Oggioni E, Pamparana F. Results of a phase IV study carried out with acipimox in type II diabetic patients with concomitant hyperlipoproteinemia. *J Int Med Res* 1989;17:373–380.

Atherosclerosis Reviews, Volume 22,
edited by A. M. Gotto, Jr. and R. Paoletti.
Raven Press, Ltd., New York © 1991.

Improvement in Atherogenic Risk Factors with Acipimox in Non–Insulin-Dependent Diabetic Subjects

R. S. Scott, C. J. Lintott, J. M. Bremer, B. Shand, and W. H. F. Sutherland

Lipid and Diabetes Research Group, Princess Margaret Hospital, Christchurch, New Zealand

Ischemic heart disease is the major cause of premature death among diabetics. Multiple factors interact to promote this enhanced atherogenicity among adult-onset diabetics. The major risk factors are hypertension, insulin resistance, lipid abnormalities, glycemic control, and hemorheological changes.

The aim of our study was to reduce the atherogenic risk among adult-onset diabetic subjects. The study approach we adopted was to use both diet and lipid-lowering therapy, measuring the atherogenic risk factors over a 36-week period. There were two phases to the study: the first was a stabilization phase of 12 weeks; the second period of 24 weeks was the treatment phase. The stabilization phase involved intensive diet counseling at 2- to 4-week intervals, with frequent medical assessments. Stringent diet targets were set: total fat $< 27\%$ of energy, saturated fat $< 8\%$ of energy, and carbohydrate $> 50\%$ of energy.

During the stabilization phase, patients were required to achieve compliance and stability of diet. Patients recruited to the treatment phase at the end of the 12-week period had to meet two biochemical criteria: fasting cholesterol levels had to lie between 5.8 mmol/L and 7.8 mmol/L, and fasting glucose levels had to be < 11.1 mmol/L. Those meeting these criteria were then randomized into one of two groups—a placebo group or a treatment group using acipimox. The treatment phase was of 24 weeks' duration.

Following randomization, patients were given one tablet (either placebo or acipimox) per day, increasing over 8 days to a total of three tablets per day. This gave the treated group 750 mg acipimox per day. Individuals were seen at 4-week intervals for dietary compliance and medical assessments. During both phases (stabilization phase and treatment phase), the following measurements were undertaken at 4- to 6-week intervals: Clinical mea-

TABLE 1. *Patient characteristics*

	Acipimox	Placebo
Sex	M, 10; F, 13	M, 9; F, 14
Age (yr)	59 (8)	60 (9)
BMI	28.5 (3.1)	27.4 (3.9)
Duration of diabetes (yr)	7.3 (4.6)	7.2 (4.6)

M = male, F = female; BMI = body mass index.

surements included nutrient analyses, measurement of body weight, body mass index (BMI), and blood pressure. Diabetes medications were also reviewed for all patients at these intervals. Biochemical measurements performed were as follows: fasting cholesterol and triglyceride (TG), apoprotein A-I and B; and high-density lipoprotein (HDL), very-low-density lipoprotein (VLDL), low-density lipoprotein (LDL), and lipoprotein (a). Glycemic control was measured by fasting glucose and glycated hemoglobin. Hemorheological parameters included fibrinogen, whole blood and plasma viscosity, red cell deformability, and red blood cell aggregation. Fasting insulin and C-peptide levels were measured at the specified times.

The patients were adult-onset diabetic subjects. We recruited 56 but lost 10 during the diet-intensive stabilization phase. This left 46 patients to enter into the trial, 23 each for the two groups (acipimox and placebo). Of the 10 lost at randomization, 8 were excluded because glycemic parameters or lipid parameters had improved to an extent with diet change that they were no longer eligible. Patient characteristics of the two randomised groups (acipimox and placebo) are shown in Table 1. Age, BMI, and duration of diabetes were evenly matched for both groups. Nine of the 23 patients in each group were on diet alone; the remainder used a variety of oral agents, singly or in combination. Wherever possible, the sulphonylurea used was standarized to glipizide.

Statistical analysis within and between (drug effect) groups were by repeated measures analysis of variance.

RESULTS

Stabilization Phase Outcomes

Given the fact that the stabilization phase was very intensive, with individuals seen in the early phases at 2- to 4-week intervals, it is not surprising that over the 12 weeks, there were marked improvements in body weights and glycemic and lipid parameters. The data at entry (-12 weeks) and at the time of randomization defined by Week 0 is shown in Tables 2 and 3. For the acipimox group, all parameters—weight, cholesterol, TG, HDL,

TABLE 2. *Diet change during stabilization phase*
(% of subjects meeting dietary targets)

	Week−12		Week 0	
	Acipimox	Placebo	Acipimox	Placebo
Total fat	31	26	78	74
Saturated fat	9	4	52	44
Cholesterol	18	22	52	65

fasting glucose, glycated Hb—improved. For the placebo group, all parameters except cholesterol changed significantly. Note the marked falls in TG levels achieved by diet intervention alone. By randomization, patients had achieved an improved and stable metabolic condition.

Treatment Phase Outcomes

Starting cholesterol values were similar for both groups. Over the 24 weeks of treatment, the acipimox-treated group sustained lower values than the placebo group. This was a significant drug effect (Fig. 1). Figure 2 shows the TG responses. At randomization, starting values were similar. Over the 24-week treatment phase, the acipimox group maintained lower values than the placebo group, although this was not significant (Fig. 2). Changes in HDL cholesterol are shown in Fig. 3. HDL levels were higher in the acipimox group than in the placebo group. This was a highly significant drug effect ($p < 0.001$).

The measured LDL cholesterol levels at Week 0 were not significantly different between the two groups. However, over the 24 weeks of treatment, LDL cholesterol levels rose significantly in the placebo group but fell in the acipimox group. As ascertained by repeated measures analysis of variance, this was a significant drug effect. VLDL triglyceride levels at Week 0 were similar. Over the 24 weeks of treatment, the trend was for values to decline in the acipimox group and to rise in the placebo group. Overall, there was

TABLE 3. *Stabilization phase outcome*

	Acipimox		Placebo	
Treatment week	− 12	0	− 12	0
Weight (kg)	78.9	78.0	76.2	74.4
Chol (mmol/L)	7.0	6.6	7.4	6.5
TG (mmol/L)	3.2	2.1	5.3	2.1
HDL (mmol/L)	1.1	1.1	1.2	1.2
FBG (mmol/L)	7.7	6.6	8.7	7.4
Glyc Hb	56.3	49.6	54.1	50.0

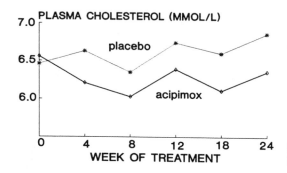

FIG. 1. Total cholesterol with acipimox treatment versus placebo.

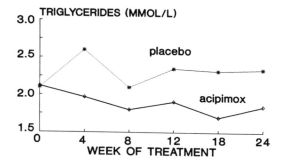

FIG. 2. Triglycerides with acipimox treatment versus placebo.

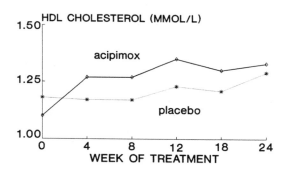

FIG. 3. HDL-cholesterol with acipimox treatment versus placebo.

TABLE 4. *Apolipoprotein B*

Treatment week	Acipimox (mg/dl)	Placebo (mg/dl)
0	120.7 (26.9)	113.4 (26.3)
12	107.5 (25.7)	115.5 (21.0)
24	97.9 (23.2)	105.3 (21.6)

Mean (SD).

TABLE 5. *Lipoprotein (a)*

Treatment week	Acipimox (mg/dl)	Placebo (mg/dl)
0	43.0 (35.7)	39.6 (37.9)
12	41.5 (37.9)	43.6 (36.6)
24	46.0 (40.0)	45.8 (42.6)

Mean (SD).

no significant drug effect. With VLDL-cholesterol, there was a significant drug effect; lower values were observed with acipimox treatment.

Table 4 shows the measured apolipoprotein B (apoB) values at Weeks 0, 12, and 24. There were no significant changes on placebo treatment. With acipimox, the 24-week values were significantly ($p < 0.001$) lower. There was a significant drug effect ($p < 0.01$). In spite of the significant increase in HDL cholesterol, there was no change for apolipoprotein A-I (apoA-I) for either group. No drug effect was observed for apolipoprotein E (apoE).

Table 5 shows lipoprotein (a) values expressed as mg/dl. There was a wide range of values at Week 0, with no significant differences between groups. No drug effect was observed. Fasting glucose values at Week 0 were not significantly different between the two groups. Although overall glycemic control was better for the acipimox than placebo group, a significant drug effect was not detected.

The acipimox group showed lower glycated hemoglobin values at Week 24 versus Week 0. Differences between the two groups as assessed by repeated measures analysis of variance did not reach statistical significance. Fasting insulin and C-peptide values were similar in both groups and no drug effect was observed. Fibrinogen levels fell significantly during acipimox treatment; this was a significant drug effect (Fig. 4). Of the various rheological parameters measured, whole blood viscosity was the only rheological parameter to show significant change. Viscosity was reduced in the acipimox-treated group. No change was noted in the placebo group. This effect

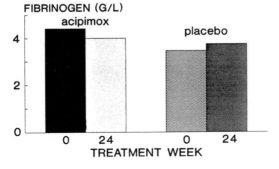

FIG. 4. Fibrinogen with acipimox treatment versus placebo.

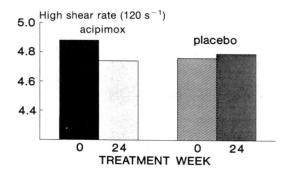

FIG. 5. Whole blood viscosity with acipimox treatment versus placebo.

of acipimox over placebo (drug effect) was significant (Fig. 5). Systolic and diastolic blood pressure values fell in both groups. There were no significant differences between the two groups.

SUMMARY

The effect of 24 weeks' acipimox treatment on atherosclerotic risk factors in diabetic subjects, tightly controlled for diet, can be summarized briefly as follows: total cholesterol fell, LDL fell, HDL rose, and apoB fell. Mean individual percentage differences at 24 weeks for acipimox versus placebo were 9% reduction for cholesterol, 8% reduction for LDL cholesterol, 30% increase for HDL, and 12% reduction in apoB. For glycemic control, there was no significant drug effect detected. However, the glycated hemoglobin values in the acipimox group did show a significant reduction between Week 0 and Week 24. Of the hemorheological parameters, fibrinogen and whole blood viscosity improved. Fibrinogen decreased 15%, and whole blood viscosity decreased 8% for the acipimox group compared with placebo.

CONCLUSION

Improvement in many of the major atherogenic risk factors present in diabetic subjects was observed with 6 months of acipimox treatment. These improvements were far greater than any that could be achieved with adherence to a strict diet program alone.

Atherosclerosis Reviews, Volume 22,
edited by A. M. Gotto, Jr. and R. Paoletti.
Raven Press, Ltd., New York © 1991.

The Action of Nicotinic Acid and Its Analogues on Lipoprotein Metabolism

James Shepherd

Institute of Biochemistry, Royal Infirmary, Glasgow G4 0SF, Scotland

Nicotinic acid amide, an essential component of the pyrimidine nucleotides, participates in a variety of oxidative reactions by acting as an electron acceptor during the dehydrogenation of specific substrates integral to the tricarboxylic acid cycle, fatty acid oxidation, the pentose phosphate pathway, etc. Although it can be generated from tryptophan, it is recognized as an essential component of a healthy diet, with a recommended daily allowance of 20 mg. When ingested in excess of requirements, it undergoes rapid urinary excretion. Large doses, however, generate an immediate antilipolytic effect that leads to short-term changes in all lipoprotein fractions in the plasma. Repeated administration of the agent produces effective and persistent lipoprotein changes that in long-term prospective studies (1,2) have been associated with reduced morbidity and mortality from coronary heart disease (CHD). These agents are therefore widely regarded as offering an effective and economical approach to CHD prevention.

Nicotinic acid and its analogues are useful in the treatment of both hypercholesterolemia and hypertriglyceridemia. Their benefits were first appreciated by Altschul et al. in 1955 (3); since then they have been prescribed with varying popularity for the treatment of all varieties of hyperlipidemia. The main drawbacks to their more widespread use are the unpleasant side effects of flushing and gastrointestinal irritation. In many subjects, these side effects can be overcome by administration of low-dose aspirin before the cholesterol-lowering drug is given. Nicotinic acid has a good safety record. Although liver enzymes may be transiently elevated in new patients, they usually return rapidly to baseline, even when the drug is continued at a lower dose. In addition to this clinical benefit, nicotinic acid should be considered because (a) it is inexpensive and, as noted above (b) it is the only lipid-lowering drug that has been shown to diminish total mortality in a clinical trial situation.

Despite 25 years of experience with nicotinic acid, many aspects of its mechanisms of action are still controversial and the subject of continuing investigation. Although some workers have used much higher levels to achieve a maximal effect, the drug is usually administered at a dose of 2 to 3 g/day (4). Virtually all of it is absorbed from the gastrointestinal tract (5), and blood levels rise to a peak within 1 hr of ingestion (6). It is nicotinic acid itself, rather than a metabolite, that appears to be the active agent; at pharmacologic doses, most of the compound is excreted unaltered into the urine (5). In an attempt to achieve the lipid-lowering while avoiding the side effects, the pharmaceutical industry has developed derivatives of nicotinic acid like acipimox that help minimize these problems and offer the clinician safer therapy at lower drug doses.

LIPID-LOWERING ACTIONS OF NICOTINIC ACID AND ITS ANALOGUES

Administration of nicotinic acid (2–3 g/day) or its recently introduced derivative acipimox (750–1,250 mg/day) produces sustained and significant reductions (up to 30–40%) in plasma triglyceride (TG) and very-low-density lipoprotein (VLDL). Although the mechanism involved is still a matter of controversy, the effect is undoubtedly associated with a profound reduction in plasma free fatty acid (FFA) levels (up to 10-fold), which is thought to diminish hepatic TG synthesis (Fig. 1) by limiting substrate availability (7).

Fat cells contain a hormone-sensitive TG lipase that in response to catecholamines increases its activity and promotes the release of fatty acids into the bloodstream. Cyclic AMP (cAMP) is believed to act as a second messenger in this hormone-induced effect. It has been shown that the cAMP concentration is reduced in fat cells exposed to nicotinic acid, possibly as a result of increased phosphodiesterase activity. This drug-induced depression of FFA release, which has been demonstrated both in isolated fat tissue and *in vivo*, appears to be the primary mode of action of the drug. There is no effect on the plasma clearance rate of FFA or on their oxidation to CO_2 during exercise. It could be predicted from the relationship between hepatic FFA uptake and VLDL TG secretion that the substantial lowering of FA levels by nicotinic acid leads to a reduced rate of VLDL production. In contrast to fibrates, there is no evidence for stimulation of lipoprotein lipase during administration of nicotinic acid.

The means by which nicotinic acid or its derivatives, such as acipimox, lowers plasma cholesterol is still not understood. There are reports of an inhibitory action of the drugs on cholesterol synthesis mediated through suppression of 3-hydroxy-3-methylglutaryl coenzyme A (HMG-CoA) reductase, but the most likely explanation for this finding is that it derives from the reduction in VLDL synthesis. A large proportion of cholesterol leaving the liver does so in the form of VLDL cholesterol. If this pathway is substantially inhibited following down-regulation of VLDL TG production, then the cholesterol that would have been secreted in the large TG-

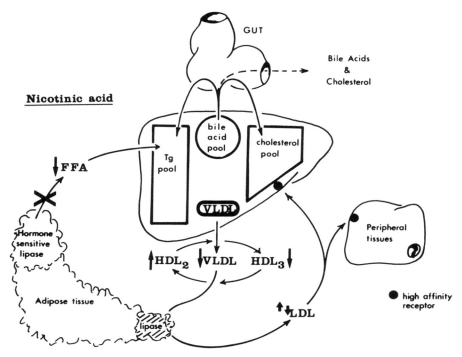

FIG. 1. Effects of nicotinic acid on lipoprotein metabolism. Nicotinic acid inhibits TG lipolysis in adipocytes and limits substrate availability for hepatic VLDL triglyceride production. VLDL secretion is therefore diminished, leading to alterations in both LDL and HDL metabolism.

rich lipoprotein (TGRLP) accumulates in the hepatocytes and may lead there to a reduction in HMG-CoA reductase levels.

Low-density lipoprotein (LDL) is variably affected by nicotinic acid analogues; as with fibrates, the final plasma concentration achieved is dependent on the initial hyperlipoproteinaemic phenotype (8,9). Subjects with high LDL starting levels experience a 10% to 15% drop in the concentration of the lipoprotein in the plasma, whereas those who have raised TG and low or subnormal LDL exhibit an increase when TG levels are reduced by the drug. Kinetic studies (10) suggest that the drug acts primarily to inhibit LDL synthesis—a finding consonant with its suppressant effect on the hepatic secretion of VLDL, the precursor of LDL. Subfractionation of LDL (d = 1.019–1.063 g/ml) by density gradient ultracentrifugation (11) yields up to four discernible classes, which have been designated LDL_1–LDL_4. In most healthy subjects, LDL_2 is the main component. Men have a higher proportion of LDL_3, the dense subfraction, whereas women have significantly higher levels of LDL_1. There is evidence to suggest that a preponderance of small, dense LDL (LDL$_3$) is associated with an increased risk of CHD (11). Treatment with acipimox induces a consistent increase in the least dense LDL subfraction (LDL$_1$) and a decrement in LDL$_3$. These changes are apparent in both normal and hyperlipidemic individuals and are accompanied by a net increase in the mean diameter of LDL particles in the circulation. It is arguable that these changes are antiatherogenic with regard to lipoprotein metabolism.

Nicotinic acid often produces marked increases in high-density lipoprotein (HDL) cholesterol (12), especially in normotriglyceridemic individuals. At the same time, there is a dramatic rise in the HDL$_2$/HDL$_3$ ratio in the plasma. Because HDL$_2$ is cardioprotective, this change is interpreted as a desirable action of the drug. Nicotinic acid alters the turnover rate of the major apolipoproteins in HDL, so that the plasma concentration of apolipoprotein (apo)A-I rises whereas that of apoA-II falls (12). Again, these changes are consonant with an increased HDL$_2$/HDL$_3$ ratio in the plasma.

COMBINED DRUG THERAPY FOR HYPERLIPIDEMIA

Therapeutic goals for plasma cholesterol and TG levels have been lowered to the extent that they supersede the effectiveness of most lipid-lowering agents. As a result, many physicians are turning to combinations of drugs in the hope that by making use of their complementary actions, they can achieve adequate control of plasma lipid and lipoprotein levels. One of the most effective combinations for cholesterol reduction (Fig. 2) is nicotinic acid or acipimox coupled with bile acid sequestrant resin therapy (13,14). This regimen can reduce total and LDL cholesterol by between 30% to 40%, even in patients with the genetic disorder familial hypercholesterolemia.

SUMMARY

Epidemiological investigations have shown that hyperlipidemia is associated with an increased risk of atherosclerosis. This risk can be reduced by treating the lipid abnormality and restoring blood cholesterol and TG levels toward normal. Although increased circulating concentrations of chylomicrons and VLDL (both TG-rich particles) do not seem to be linked to the atherosclerotic process directly, they may predispose the sufferer to this condition as a result of their negative association with the protective lipoprotein fraction, HDL. Cholesterol-rich particles—particularly remnants of VLDL metabolism—and LDL itself seem to be especially atherogenic. Nicotinic acid and its analogues produce beneficial effects on all of the above plasma lipoprotein fractions. The circulating mass of VLDL and LDL falls during therapy while HDL levels (particularly the antiatherogenic HDL$_2$ fraction) rise. It is arguable, on the basis of our understanding of lipoprotein

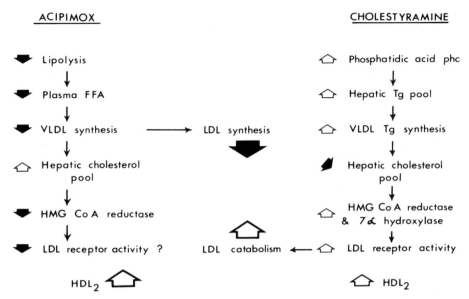

FIG. 2. Combined lipid-lowering actions of acipimox and cholestyramine. Acipimox and cholestyramine resin exert complementary actions on lipoprotein metabolism that offer particular benefits in the treatment of combined hypercholesterolemia and hypertriglyceridemia. Acipimox limits substrate availability for hepatic VLDL production, blunting the potentially hypertriglyceridemic actions of the resin. In addition, a significant reduction of plasma LDL is to be expected as a result of inhibition of its synthesis by acipimox and promotion of its catabolism by cholestyramine. Both drugs raise plasma HDL by mechanisms that are not yet completely understood.

metabolism, that these actions in aggregate offer overall cardioprotection to the recipient.

REFERENCES

1. Coronary Drug Project. Clofibrate and niacin in coronary heart disease. *JAMA* 1975;231:360–381.
2. Blankenhorn DH, Nessim SA, Johnson RL, et al. Beneficial effects of combined colestipol and niacin therapy on coronary atherosclerosis and coronary venous bypass grafts. *J Am Med Assoc* 1987;257:3233–3240.
3. Altschul R, Hoffer A, Stephen JD. Influence of nicotinic acid on serum cholesterol in man. *Arch Biochem Biophys* 1955;54:558–559.
4. Lewis B. The hyperlipidaemias. Oxford: Blackwell Scientific Publishers, 1976:356.
5. Miller ON, Hamilton JG, Goldsmith GA. Investigation of the mechanism of action of nicotinic acid on serum lipid levels in man. *Am J Clin Nutr* 1960;8:480–490.
6. Fumagalli R. Pharmacokinetics of nicotinic acid and some of its derivatives. In: Gey KF, Carlson LA, eds. *Metabolic effects of nicotinic acid and its derivatives.* Bern–New York: Hans Huber, 1971:33.
7. Carlson LA, Oro L. The effect of nicotinic acid on plasma free fatty acids. Demonstration of a metabolic type of sympathicolysis. *Acta Med Scand* 1962;172:641–645.

8. Carlson LA, Oro L, Ostman J. Effect of nicotinic acid on plasma lipids in patients with hyperlipoproteinemia during the first week of treatment. *Atherosclerosis* 1968;8:667–677.
9. Carlson LA, Olsson AG, Ballantyne D. On the rise in LDL and HDL in response to the treatment of hypertriglyceridaemia in Type IV and Type V hyperlipoproteinemias. *Atherosclerosis* 1977;26:603–609.
10. Levy RI, Langer T. Hypolipidemic drugs and lipoprotein metabolism. *Adv Exp Med Biol* 1972;26:155–163.
11. Griffin BA, Caslake MJ, Yip B, Tait GW, Packard CJ, Shepherd J. Rapid isolation of discrete LDL subfractions from plasma by density gradient ultracentrifugation. *Atherosclerosis* 1990;83:59–67.
12. Shepherd J, Packard CJ, Patsch JR, Gotto AM, Taunton OD. Effect of nicotinic acid on plasma HDL subfraction distribution and composition and on apolipoprotein A metabolism. *J Clin Invest* 1979;63:858–867.
13. Packard CJ, Stewart JM, Morgan HG, Lorimer AR, Shepherd J. Combined drug therapy for familial hypercholesterolemia. *Artery* 1980;7:281–289.
14. Series JJ, Gaw A, Kilday C, et al. Acipimox in combination with low dose cholestyramine for the treatment of type II hyperlipidaemia. *Br J Clin Pharmacol* 1990;30:49–54.

Atherosclerosis Reviews, Volume 22,
edited by A. M. Gotto, Jr. and R. Paoletti.
Raven Press, Ltd., New York © 1991.

Effects of Acipimox on Plasma Lipoproteins of Hyperlipidemic Human Subjects

P. J. Barter, L. Nelson, S. Devlin, and P. Jenkins

Baker Medical Research Institute, Australia

A study of the effects of acipimox on plasma lipoproteins was performed in 18 subjects (15 male and 3 female) with mixed hyperlipidemia of type IIb phenotype in whom the plasma cholesterol was 6.0 to 9.0 mM and the plasma triglyceride (TG) was 2.0 to 8.0 mM. The study was an open design without placebo or active controls. Following a 3-month run-in period when treatment was limited to a lipid-lowering diet, subjects were treated for 6 months with acipimox at a dose of 250 mg three times daily.

Plasma samples collected immediately prior to commencing acipimox and after 3 and 6 months of treatment were subjected to detailed lipid and lipoprotein analysis. Whole plasma was assayed for cholesterol, TG, and apolipoproteins A-I, A-II, and B (apoA-I, apoA-II, apoB, respectively). Very-low-density lipoproteins (VLDL) were isolated by ultracentrifugation and assayed for cholesterol, TG, phospholipid, apoA, and total protein. The low-density lipoproteins (LDL) and high-density lipoproteins (HDL) were separated for the plasma fraction of density (d) > 1.006 g/ml. This fraction was first subjected to ultracentrifugation at d = 1.25 g/ml to remove the bulk of the nonlipoprotein proteins. The LDL and HDL in the fraction of 1.006 to 1.25 g/ml were then separated by size exclusion chromatography on a column of Superose 6 HR 10/30 attached to a high-pressure pump (1). Multiple fractions were collected and assayed for lipid and apolipoprotein constituents. The fractions containing LDL were identified by the distribution of apoB; those containing HDL were identified by the distribution of apoA-I. There was very little overlap between the LDL and HDL. The fractions containing LDL and those containing HDL were each combined to determine lipoprotein concentrations and compositions. Recoveries of cholesterol in the LDL and HDL after this separation were about 85% of that in the plasma fraction of d > 1.006 g/ml; values have been corrected for recovery. The lipoprotein compositions were determined after assaying for cholesterol, TG, apoB, apoA-I and, apoA-II. The protein content of LDL was taken as the apoB content; the protein content of HDL was taken as the sum of apoA-I and apoA-II.

To determine the particle size distribution of LDL and HDL, samples of plasma were subjected to ultracentrifugation at d = 1.25 g/ml; the supernatant was recovered and separated by nondenaturing polyacrylamide gel electrophoresis on 2% to 16% gradient gels for LDL and 4% to 30% gradient gels for HDL (2,3). After electrophoresis, gels were fixed, stained, and scanned by a laser densitometer that was attached to an integrator for quantitating the relative proportions of the different subpopulations. The particle size of LDL has been defined in terms of the radius (nm) of the major population. The subpopulation distribution of HDL has been calculated as the percentage of the total HDL that exist as HDL_2, HDL_{3a} and HDL_{3b} subpopulations. The data were analyzed using standard analysis of variance procedures for repeated measurements.

RESULTS

Concentration of Constituents in Whole Plasma

The concentration of plasma TG was reduced by 34.2% ($p > 0.001$) after 3 months of treatment with acipimox. After 6 months, the reduction was 36.3% ($p < 0.001$). A reduction in the concentration of plasma cholesterol was less apparent but also significant; after 6 months, the plasma cholesterol was reduced by 8.9% ($p < 0.05$). The concentration of plasma apoB was reduced by 10.9% ($p < 0.01$) after 3 months and by 9.9% ($p < 0.01$) after 6 months of therapy with acipimox. By contrast, there were no significant changes in the plasma concentrations of either apoA-I or apoA-II.

Concentration of Lipoprotein Fractions

The concentration of VLDL TG was reduced by 36.4% after 3 months ($p < 0.01$) and by 35.8% after 6 months ($p < 0.01$) of acipimox therapy. The VLDL cholesterol was reduced by 50.6% at 3 months ($p < 0.001$) and by 51.5% after 6 months of therapy ($p < 0.001$). The concentration of VLDL apoB was reduced by 40.8% at 3 months ($p < 0.001$) and by 38.3% at 6 months ($p < 0.001$).

The concentration of LDL cholesterol was unchanged at both the 3-month and the 6-month visits. Likewise, there was no significant change in the concentration of LDL apoB at either visit. There was, however, a reduction of the LDL TG concentration of 28.2% at 3 months ($p < 0.01$) and 31.0% at 6 months ($p < 0.01$).

The concentration of HDL cholesterol was increased by 10.4% at 3 months ($p < 0.05$) and by 7.6% at 6 months ($p < 0.05$). The HDL TG concentration was reduced by 26.3% at 3 months ($p < 0.05$) and by 36.8% at 6 months ($p < 0.05$). The concentrations of HDL apoA-I and apoA-II did not change.

Composition of Lipoprotein Fractions

Coinciding with the reductions in the concentration of VLDL constituents, there were significant changes in the composition of VLDL. The cholesterol content of VLDL decreased from 13.8% before acipimox to 10.3% after 6 months ($p < 0.01$). There was concurrent increase in the TG content of VLDL from 58.3% pre-acipimox to 63.3% at 6 months ($p < 0.01$). The mass ratio of TG/cholesterol in VLDL increased dramatically from 4.60 before acipimox to 6.23 at 3 months ($p < 0.001$) and 6.43 at 6 months ($p < 0.001$).

Although changes in the composition of LDL were much smaller, they were significant in the case of phospholipid, which increased from 25.6% before acipimox to 27.2% after 6 months ($p < 0.001$), and protein, which decreased from 20.0% to 19.4% after 6 months ($p < 0.01$). Changes in the LDL composition of cholesterol and TG were not significant.

The only significant change in composition of HDL was a reduction of TG content from 5.4% before acipimox to 3.9% after 6 months ($p < 0.05$).

Particle Size Distribution of Lipoproteins

The particle size of LDL increased after acipimox. Gradient gel electrophoresis revealed that the radius of the major LDL population increased from a mean of 12.3 nm before acipimox to 12.7 nm after 6 months ($p < 0.05$). In 10 normolipidemic subjects, the mean radius of the major LDL population was 12.9 nm.

There were also changes in the particle size distribution of HDL after acipimox; however, the response was variable and involved mainly the HDL_3 subfraction. Most of the subjects had no measurable HDL_2 before therapy with acipimox; treatment had little or no effect on this fraction. Thus, as a percentage of the total HDL, HDL_2 accounted for a mean of only 2.7% before acipimox, 2.8% after 3 months, and 3.9% after 6 months. In the case of HDL_3, there was a relative increase in the proportion of the subpopulation of the larger HDL_{3a} particles from a mean of 54.8% before acipimox to 60.2% after 6 months; however, this change was not statistically significant. There was a relative decrease in the proportion of the subpopulation of smaller HDL_{3b} particles from a mean of 42.5% and 35.8% after 6 months ($p < 0.05$). In 15 normolipidemic subjects, HDL_2, HDL_{3a}, and HDL_{3b} accounted for 15%, 65%, and 20%, respectively, of the total HDL.

Adverse Events

There were no serious adverse events and all 18 subjects completed the study. Although mild flushing occurred in 12 subjects, it only lasted for a few days despite continuing therapy. Two individuals developed a skin rash; it was mild in one and moderate in the other. One subject reported occasional mild nausea during the 1st month, and another experienced mild itchiness that lasted for 3 days during the 1st month. There was no evidence of hepatotoxicity.

CONCLUSIONS

This study corroborates many previous observations that acipimox at a dose of 750 mg/day is a highly effective agent for treating hypertriglyceridemia in patients with the common disorder of combined hyperlipidemia (type IIb phenotype). The results also reveal additional effects of acipimox in modifying plasma lipoproteins toward a less atherogenic profile. These positive effects include increase in HDL cholesterol, increase in the particle size distribution of both HDL and LDL, and—most dramatically—a reduction in the cholesterol content of the VLDL fraction. The latter finding is a strong indication of a reduction in the concentration of atherogenic remnant lipoproteins. Acipimox was well tolerated by the subjects, who remained free of serious side effects.

REFERENCES

1. Clay MA, Hopkins GJ, Ehnholm CP, Barter PJ. The rabbit as an animal model of hepatic lipase deficiency. *Biochim Biophys Acta* 1989;1002:173–181.
2. Blanch PJ, Gong EL, Forte TM, Nichols AV. Characterization of human high-density lipoproteins by gradient gel electrophoresis. *Biochim Biophys Acta* 1981;665:408–419.
3. Krauss RM, Burke DJ. Identification of multiple subclasses of plasma low density lipoproteins. *J Lipid Res* 1982;23:97–104.

Atherosclerosis Reviews, Volume 22,
edited by A. M. Gotto, Jr. and R. Paoletti.
Raven Press, Ltd., New York © 1991.

Long-Term Safety Profile of Acipimox

Pharmacological Basis and Clinical Evidence

B. M. Buckley

Department of Endocrinology and Metabolism, Bon Secours Hospital, Cork, Ireland

For more than 30 years, nicotinic acid has been widely used in the treatment of hypercholesterolemia and hypertriglyceridemia. Although it is regarded as a safe and effective drug, nicotinic acid suffers from a number of major disadvantages that have limited its use in clinical practice. Foremost is the fact that it causes a cutaneous nonhistaminic flush reaction that is sometimes severe and may be associated with pruritus before steady-state plasma concentrations are achieved. In addition, hyperglycemia occurs due to inhibition of glucose catabolism because suppressed nonesterified fatty acid (NEFA) concentrations rebound when plasma nicotinic acid concentrations decline after dosing. Because of its short plasma elimination half-life, dose intervals have to be short in order to attain steady state, avoid these adverse reactions, and achieve therapeutic efficacy.

Acipimox (5-methylpyramine-2-carboxylic-4-oxide) is an isoster of 5-methyl-nicotinic acid-M-oxide. It is more effective than nicotinic acid in causing plasma cholesterol and triglyceride (TG) concentrations to decrease, and its plasma elimination half-life is longer. Because of these properties, cutaneous flushing is diminished, and the drug can be administered twice or three times daily. The flush response can be suppressed with aspirin.

Studies in Italy, Germany, and the United Kingdom have investigated the long-term safety, tolerability, and efficacy of acipimox (as Olbetam) in routine clinical practice. The results indicate that the drug decreases plasma concentrations of TG as well as total and low-density lipoprotein (LDL) cholesterol while increasing high-density lipoprotein (HDL) cholesterol. As expected, cutaneous flushing is the principal adverse effect encountered. Headache and gastrointestinal disturbance are reported less frequently. A small number of cases of serious adverse reactions following first exposure to acipimox have been reported; the features of these reactions suggest the possibility of type I immediate hypersensitivity reaction. No fatalities have been recorded. Acipimox has not been found to adversely affect hepatic or renal function or hematopoiesis.

PHARMACOKINETICS OF ACIPIMOX IN HUMANS

Acipimox is absorbed rapidly from the human gastrointestinal tract following oral dosing. In single-dose volunteer studies (1), peak plasma levels are generally achieved within 2 hr of administration and are linearly related to the size of the dose administered, as is the area under the concentration-time curve (AUC). Acipimox is water-soluble and does not bind to human albumin *in vitro*. It has an apparent volume of distribution of the order of 30 liters. Acipimox is eliminated by the kidneys without appreciable biotransformation; it has a mean initial plasma elimination half-life ($T_{1/2}$) of about 2 hr. After approximately 8 hr, the rate of elimination from plasma slows to about one-sixth of this. About 90% of the administered dose appears unchanged in urine after 24 hr. However, the conversion of small amounts of acipimox to 5-methylpyrazine-carboxylic acid has been observed in animals and in some human subjects, almost certainly through the action of the gut flora in the distal intestine. Concomitant food ingestion with acipimox dosing slows the absorption of the drug, more than doubling T_{max}, but does not significantly alter AUC, C_{max}, or $T_{1/2}$ (1).

Administration of cholestyramine concomitantly with acipimox did not have any significant effect on acipimox plasma concentrations or on any major pharmacokinetic characteristic of acipimox (2). The pharmacokinetic behavior of the drug after a single dose is summarized in Table 1. Repeated dosing until steady-state conditions are reached causes an increase in C_{max} and in AUC (6.0 mg/L and 23 mg/L/hr, respectively, for 250 mg three times daily; see Table 1 for comparison); but there is no evidence of accumulation, and in the presence of normal renal function, a three-times-daily dose schedule is appropriate (Farmitalia Carlo Erba, Ltd., unpublished data). By contrast to acipimox, nicotinic acid has a $T_{1/2}$ of less than 1 hr (3). Thus it requires very short dose intervals to achieve steady-state conditions and avoid wide fluctuations in plasma concentrations.

Because acipimox is cleared from plasma principally by renal excretion, its plasma elimination in patients with renal impairment is slower than in healthy subjects; $T_{1/2}$ becomes progressively longer as creatinine clearance decreases. At creatinine clearances of 10 to 30 ml/min, $T_{1/2}$ increases to about

TABLE 1. *Single-dose pharmacokinetic characteristics of acipimox[a]*

	Dose		
	150 mg	250 mg	400 mg
C_{max} (mg/L)	1.8 ± 0.5	3.6 ± 0.4	5.0 ± 1.3
T_{max} (hr)	1.8 ± 0.5	1.8 ± 0.5	1.5 ± 0.6
$AUC_{0-32\ hr}$ (mg/L/hr)	9.3	16.7	29.4

[a] Data from ref. 1.

5.2 hr to 8.0 hr (3). The pharmacokinetics of acipimox in elderly subjects are determined largely by their renal function.

PHARMACODYNAMICS

The most immediate observed effect of acipimox on lipid metabolism *in vivo* is to decrease plasma NEFA concentrations. It is about six times more active than nicotinic acid on a mg/kg body weight basis (4,5). As with nicotinic acid, this effect results from inhibition of catecholamine-stimulated lipolysis in adipose tissue (6,7, and unpublished data of Farmitalia Carlo Erba, Ltd.), probably through activation of adipocyte membrane high-affinity GTPase, an allosteric enzyme at the regulatory site of adenylate cyclase (7). Lipolysis is thereby decreased, causing plasma NEFA concentrations to fall and decreasing their flux to the liver. As a result, less NEFA is available as substrate for hepatic TG and very-low-density lipoprotein (VLDL) synthesis, decreasing plasma VLDL concentrations. Consequently, LDL synthesis is decreased, and plasma HDL concentrations are increased. The antilipolytic activity of acipimox in humans is greater, in terms both of dose response and duration of effect, than that of nicotinic acid.

Acipimox also enhances the activity of adipose tissue lipoprotein lipase, the rate-limiting enzyme in the catabolism of VLDL in plasma (unpublished data, Farmitalia Carlo Erba, Ltd.). It is not clear whether this effect makes a significant contribution to the lipid-lowering action of acipimox. Acipimox has no effect on the activity of HMG-CoA reductase or the rate of cholesterol synthesis in rat liver or intestinal slices (unpublished data, Farmitalia Carlo Erba, Ltd.) or in human jejunal mucosa *in vitro* (6).

Fibric acid derivatives cause considerable hepatic peroxisomal proliferation. However, acipimox has no effect on peroxisome enzymes; instead, it causes a decrease in fatty acid β-oxidation (8,9).

ACIPIMOX TOXICOLOGY IN ANIMALS

The usual therapeutic dose of acipimox in humans is 750 mg/day, which is equivalent to about 10 mg/kg of body weight per day. Doses of 15 mg/kg of body weight per day are occasionally used. The maximum likely therapeutic dose of acipimox in humans is about 30 mg/kg of body weight per day. Acipimox is of low acute toxicity in animal studies. The minimum single dose LD_{50} exceeds 1,900 mg/kg of body weight in the most susceptible mouse strain and 2,000 mg/kg of body weight in the most susceptible strains of rat and dog (unpublished data, Farmitalia Carlo Erba, Ltd.). These values are comparable to those known for nicotinic acid (4). In 13-week subacute studies, the no-adverse-effect levels (NOAEL) observed in mice, rats, and dogs were respectively 2,700, 400, and 810 mg/kg of body weight per day (unpublished data, Farmitalia Carlo Erba, Ltd.). Although hemorrhagic lesions were observed in the upper alimentary tract in the high-dose acute LD_{50} studies, no such lesions were reported in the 13-week subacute studies (unpublished data, Farmitalia Carlo Erba, Ltd.). In long-term safety studies, the NOAEL for rats treated over 12 months was 900 mg/kg of body weight per day. Dogs were susceptible to drug-related emesis, but they tolerated a dose of 400 mg/kg of body weight per day in a 6-month study and the top dose of 900 mg/kg of body weight per day in the 24-month study. Importantly, further studies showed that the drug had no reproductive toxicity and was neither carcinogenic nor mutagenic. It had no effect on the structure or integrity of the ocular lens. These data show that there is, at a conservative estimate, a 10-fold safety factor between the minimum toxic doses in animals and the highest therapeutic doses likely to be used in humans.

ACIPIMOX: TOLERABILITY IN HUMANS

Just as acipimox and nicotinic acid share the same mechanism of action and have qualitatively similar effects on plasma lipids, they have closely similar adverse effects—principally cutaneous flushing, pruritus, urticaria, heartburn, nausea, gastrointestinal irritation, and headache.

The nonhistaminic cutaneous flush reaction appears to be prostaglandin-mediated. It seems to depend less on the absolute dose administered than on a rapid increase in plasma concentration from a low initial level. Tolerance develops in most subjects once steady-state plasma concentrations are attained. Because of the short $T_{1/2}$ of nicotinic acid, steady state is attained with difficulty when convenient dose schedules are used, and the flushing often persists to some extent. This side effect represents a serious impediment to compliance. The fact that it is easier to achieve steady-state plasma drug concentrations using smaller doses of acipimox results in a significantly lower incidence of flushing and a more rapid development of tolerance than occurs with nicotinic acid.

Twelve reports have been published describing severe angioedema and anaphylactoid reactions associated with acipimox use (unpublished data, Farmitalia Carlo Erba, Ltd.). Ten patients were participants in clinical trials or in postmarketing surveillance, and all of them experienced the reaction with the initial dose. The reactions characteristically took the form of urticaria, mucosal edema, dyspnea, and hypotension. One of these events was considered life-threatening by the attending physician, but the patient was apparently not hospitalized. Three patients had a serious reaction. Nine required medication for the attack, mainly corticosteroids and/or antihistamines. Three patients who were subsequently given acipimox again had the same reaction. Although there have been four other reports of similar reactions, they are too poorly documented to allow adequate assessment.

At present, it is difficult to define the true incidence of these reactions to acipimox. The incidence in trials and in postmarketing surveillance is about 1/1,000. However, the incidence is nontrial, nonsurveyed routine open prescription use is about one in 100,000 recipients.

The gastrointestinal effects of nicotinic acid are partly attributable to the direct irritant effect of a weak acid ($pK_a \sim 3.5$) on the upper gastrointestinal tract. Five patients in whom preexisting peptic ulcer disease was activated by very high doses of nicotinic acid (3.0–7.5 g/day) enjoyed resolution of their symptoms when this drug was administered in a buffered preparation (10). It is possible that some of the gastrointestinal irritation may also be due to the acidity of acipimox, which in 0.5% aqueous solution has a pH of 1.6 to 2.6. A major problem with nicotinic acid has been a concomitant deterioration in glucose tolerance. This effect, which was noted soon after the drug's introduction and has been confirmed many times since then (11–15), is associated with a rapid rebound and overshoot in plasma NEFA levels as plasma concentrations of nicotinic acid fall. It is probably a direct effect of NEFA on the glucose–fatty acid cycle. In contrast, acipimox administration does not adversely affect plasma glucose concentrations or insulin resistance in non–insulin-dependent diabetic patients (NIDDM); rather, it improves glucose tolerance (16).

Another adverse effect of nicotinic acid is a consistent increase in plasma urate concentrations and uric acid excretion. Chronic use of the drug increases the incidence of acute gouty arthritis (14,15,17). However, acipimox does not appear to cause this problem, as evidenced from observation of patients in trials and postmarketing surveillance studies.

Fibric acid derivatives and particularly clofibrate may alter the lithogenicity of bile and cause cholelithiasis. Acipimox administration has no significant adverse effect on bile composition (18). It may in fact decrease bile lithogenicity by lowering bile cholesterol concentration without changing phospholipid or bile acid concentrations (19).

EFFICACY IN HYPERLIPIDEMIC PATIENTS

In controlled trials conducted in several countries using a large number of hyperlipidemic patients, acipimox caused a statistically significant decrease, compared with baseline, in plasma TG concentrations of the order of 25% to 45%. On average, it decreased plasma cholesterol concentrations by 10% to 15% and increased plasma HDL cholesterol levels by about 10%.

These findings were confirmed by long-term postmarketing surveillance studies that showed similar changes in plasma lipid levels during acipimox treatment (Table 2) (20–22, and unpublished data, Farmitalia Carlo Erba, Ltd.).

TABLE 2. *Efficacy of acipimox shown in postmarketing surveillance trials*

	Study no.			
	1[a]	2[b]	3[c]	4[d]
No. of subjects	3,993	3,009	344	1,434
Duration (mo)	24	2	12	24
Δ Triglyceride %	−40	−43	−24	−19
Δ Cholesterol %	−23	−18	−7	−12
Δ HDL %	+4	+15	+20	+13

[a] From ref. 20.
[b] From ref. 21.
[c] From ref. 22.
[d] Unpublished data, Farmitalia Carlo Erba, Ltd.

ACIPIMOX: LONG-TERM SAFETY

Data have been collected on over 13,000 patients treated with acipimox for at least 1 year. The adverse effects were the same as those previously noted in earlier controlled trials (see Table 3). Tolerance to cutaneous effects such as pruritus and flushing almost always developed after a few days. In some centers, aspirin was used to block the flush reaction until tolerance developed. Most of the adverse reactions were rated as mild. There was a generally inverse relationship between the frequency and severity of adverse effects and the duration of therapy. Acipimox caused no effects on hematological or biochemical parameters that might indicate toxicity. A few adverse effects were rated as severe; these included urticarial and angioedematous reactions. No deaths were associated with an adverse reaction to the drug. Notably, mean plasma glucose concentrations were unaffected by acipimox, while plasma urate concentrations tended to fall slightly.

TABLE 3. *Acipimox: adverse effects*

	Study no.			
	1[a]	2[b]	3[c]	4[d]
No. of subjects	7,447	3,009	344	1,641
Duration (mo)	24	2	12	24
% With adverse effects	16	8.8	10	15
% Cutaneous	9.8	5.1	10	9.4
% Gastrointestinal	6.3	2.2	3	6.3
% Nervous & others	0	0.9	0.8	4.3
% Withdrawn	4.9	5.5	7.5	7

[a] From ref. 20.
[b] From ref. 21.
[c] From ref. 22.
[d] Unpublished data, Farmitalia Carlo Erba, Ltd.

CONCLUSIONS

Acipimox lowers plasma cholesterol and TG concentrations and increases plasma HDL cholesterol levels to a greater degree than nicotinic acid but via a similar mechanism. Its effect on plasma lipid levels is of similar magnitude to the fibric acid derivatives currently prescribed. Its longer persistence in plasma allows a conventional three-times-daily dose regimen and avoids the major adverse metabolic complications of glucose intolerance and hyperuricemia that occur with nicotinic acid. Instead, it has a beneficial effect on these parameters. A further effect of its longer plasma elimination half-life is that tolerance to the troublesome cutaneous flush reaction, which is associated with rapidly rising plasma drug concentrations, develops more rapidly. Apart from a low incidence of severe hypersensitivity reactions, the drug has proven to be of low toxicity in the long term. Acipimox is therefore an important addition to the pharmacopia of lipid-lowering agents.

ACKNOWLEDGMENTS

I am grateful to Farmitalia Carlo Erba, Ltd., for permission to study and refer to their data. The opinions and interpretations in this paper are the author's and do not necessarily reflect those of Farmitalia Carlo Erba, Ltd.

REFERENCES

1. Musatti L, Maggi E, Moro E, et al. Bioavailability and pharmacokinetics in man of acipimox, a new antilipolytic and hypolipemic agent. *J Int Med Res* 1981;9:381–386.
2. DePaolis C, Farina R, Pianezzola E, et al. Lack of pharmacokinetic interaction between cholestyramine and acipimox, a new lipid lowering agent. *Br J Clin Pharmacol* 1986;22:496–497.
3. Hotz W. Nicotinic acid and its derivatives: a short survey. *Adv Lipid Res* 1983;20:195–217.
4. Ambrogi V, Cozzi P, Sanjust P, et al. Antilipolytic effect of a series of pyrazine-N-oxides. *Eur J Med Chem/Chim Ther* 1980;15:157–163.
5. Lovisolo PP, Briatico-Vangosa G, Orsini G, et al. Pharmacological profile of a new antilipolytic agent: 5-methyl-pyrazine-2-carboxylic acid oxide (acipimox). 2. Antilipolytic and blood lipid lowering activity. *Pharmacol Res Commun* 1981;13:163–174.
6. Stirling M, McAleen M, Reckless JPD, et al. Effects of acipimox, a nicotinic acid derivative, on lipolysis in human adipose tissue and on cholesterol synthesis in human jejunal mucosa. *Clin Sci* 1985;68:83–88.
7. Astories LK, Schultz G, Jacobs KH. Inhibition of acenylate cyclase and stimulation of a high-affinity GTPase by the antilipolytic agents nicotinic acid, acipimox and various related compounds. *Arzneimittelforschung* 1983;33:1525–1527.
8. Locci Cubbedu T, Bergamini E. Effects of antilipolytic agents on peroxisomal beta-oxidation of fatty acids in rat liver. *Biochem Pharmacol* 1983;32:1807–1809.
9. Locci Cubbedu T, Bergamini E. Antilipolytic agents can affect the peroxisomal oxidation of fatty acids in rat liver. *Bull Mol Biol Med* 1982;7:47–54.
10. Parsons WB. Activation of peptic ulcer by nicotinic acid. *JAMA* 1960;173:92–96.
11. Gurian H, Adlersberg D. The effect of large doses of nicotinic acid on circulating lipids and carbohydrate tolerance. *Am J Med Sci* 1959;237:12–22.

12. Molnar GD, Berge KG, Rosevear JW, et al. The effect of nicotinic acid in diabetes mellitus. *Metabolism* 1964;13:181–189.
13. Miettinen TA, Taskinen MR, Pelkonen R, Nikkila EA. Glucose tolerance and plasma insulin in man during acute and chronic administration of nicotinic acid. *Acta Med Scand* 1969;186:247–253.
14. Gaur ZN, Pocelinko R, Solomon HM, Thomas GB. Oral glucose tolerance, plasma insulin and uric acid excretion in man during chronic administration of nicotinic acid. *Metabolism* 1971;20:1031–1035.
15. Garg A, Grundy SM. Nicotinic acid as therapy for dyslipidemia in non–insulin-dependent diabetes mellitus. *JAMA* 1990;264:723–726.
16. Dulbecco A, Albenga C, Borreta G, et al. Effect on plasma glucose levels in patients with non–insulin-dependent diabetes mellitus. *Curr Therapeutic Res* 1989;46:478–483.
17. Coronary Drug Project Research Group. Clofibrate and niacin in coronary heart disease. *JAMA* 1975;231:360–381.
18. Jung W, Kohlmeier M. Nikolaus TH, et al. Effects of acipimox on plasma lipids and biliary lipids in healthy subjects. *Res Exp Med* 1985;185:457–468.
19. Ericsson S, Ericsson M, Angelin B. Acipimox therapy and biliary lipids. Effects of short-term treatment in patients with combined hyperlipoproteinaemia. (in press)
20. Luley C, Krueger KJ, Schumacher M, Reider HP, Kaplan E, Kloer HU. Plasma lipids in 6255 hyperlipidemic patients upon treatment with acipimox (Olbemox) for two years. Presented at the International Symposium "Triglycerides. The Role in Diabetes and Atherosclerosis," Vienna, May 1990.
21. Lavezzari M, Milanesi E, Oggioni E, Pamparana F. Results of a phase IV study carried out with acipimox in type II diabetic patients with concomitant hyperlipidaemia. *J Int Med Res* 1989;17:373–380.
22. Muggeo M, Lavezzari M, Montoro C, et al. Long-term multicentre trial with acipimox in diabetic patients with hyperlipoproteinemia. In: Lenzi S, Descovich GC, eds. *Atherosclerosis and cardiovascular diseases*. Lancaster: MTP Press, 1987:459–472.

Subject Index